The Control of the Mind

British Library Cataloguing-in-Publication Data
A catalogue record for this book is available from the
British Library

The Control of the Mind *A HANDBOOK OF APPLIED PSYCHOLOGY FOR THE ORDINARY MAN. BY ROBERT H. THOULESS, M.A., PH.D.*

Contents

THERE are certain Indian ascetics, called Yogis, who practise a systematic development of their minds at the end of which they claim to be able to think about one thing alone or even to empty their minds of all thought. A particular kind of Yoga, called Hatha-Yoga, claims to produce in its followers perfect health and an ability to go on living indefinitely. It is claimed that it can produce even more remarkable results than this, and I have met an Indian student who assured me that he had often seen an old Yogi fly. It sounds surprising, but my informant was very certain about it.

The Buddhist ascetics practise an arduous system of thinking about the causes of desire and about life and death generally, which is supposed to result in the extinction of all desire and in the ability to keep the mind unoccupied by any thought whatever.

St. Ignatius Loyola has handed down to

us what are called the " spiritual exercises "
—a system of meditation which had as its
aim the strengthening of the religious senti-
ment. This has been the model on which
most Christian systems of religious meditation
have been founded.

Monsieur Coué teaches us to get rid of
diseases by a method of auto-suggestion,
which takes the form of repeating sentences
to ourselves. He would have us say twenty
times every night and morning : " Day by
day, in every way, I am getting better and
better."

All of these things—the Yoga systems,
religious meditation and auto-suggestion—
are what we may call *mental exercises.*
They have very different aims, but they are
all alike attempts to control the development of the mind in just the same way as
dumb-bells control the development of the
body. They are a kind of dumb-bells of
the mind. Some of them are very strenuous,
and would require the greater part of a
lifetime to produce any results.

But mental exercises are not confined to
these rather unusual things. Whenever we
carry out any task of concentrated learning we
are as truly exercising our minds as if we were

practising concentration by the method of the Yogis. Provided that the object of our learning is not that we want to be able to recall the particular thing learnt, but that we want to train our capacity for attention, we are as truly carrying out a mental exercise as a person who lifts a weight for the sake of developing his muscles is carrying out a physical exercise. A school child engaged in learning poetry, performing geometrical and algebraical puzzles, and so on, is carrying out a systematic course of mental exercises to fit his mind for the tasks it will have to perform when he has grown up.

Most of us give up the practice of mental exercising after we leave school, presumably because we are satisfied that our minds perform all the tasks that we demand of them to our complete satisfaction. If we are right in this conviction there is certainly no reason why we should bother ourselves with our mental development after our school days are over, but are we right? Do we never show any of the symptoms of mental inefficiency—worry, mind wandering, irritability, depression, or needless fears? The ideal of further mental development should not appear childish or futile to the

11

adult who is not free from these things. Psychology may still have something of practical usefulness to teach him.

Of course, normal people do not bother about their mental development. In truth, not very many normal people do physical exercises with dumb-bells at all systematically. Still fewer do any systematic exercises for their minds.

It does not appear to be true, however, that ordinary people are not interested in these things. A large number of methods are put forward which are claimed to make people happier, wiser and even wealthier, and anyone who announces that he is going to communicate such a system by means of a lecture can fill a large hall and arouse a good deal of enthusiasm amongst his hearers even if they do not systematically carry his precepts into practice. The lecturer, at least, can become wealthier, even if his audience are no happier or wiser.

Such a speaker is sometimes a man of rare and peculiar gifts. He may, however, have no qualification for guiding other people, except the doubtful quality of being able to carry conviction by a confident manner of delivery. It is quite likely that he has nothing to tell his hearers which they could not have found out for themselves by consulting ordinary textbooks on psychology, such, for example, as William James's book on *The Principles of Psychology*, which may be found in any public library.

Of course this does not mean that the lecturer serves no useful purpose, because many people learn things by personal contact that they would never take the trouble to find out for themselves from books. But when such lecturers take high fees from people who can obviously not afford to pay them, and often give in return little but high-sounding promises, we cannot regard them as socially useful.

Why do people go to lectures which claim to tell them how to " overcome their limitations," to give them " a master-key to mental success," or " mastery of the world through self-knowledge," and why do they buy books entitled " Concentration," " Self-knowledge " or something of that kind? I suppose the answer is that the people amongst whom this demand exists suspect that their minds are not working at their fullest possible efficiency.

No doubt they are often right. They suffer

from worry, from mental inertia, from irritability and timidity, from sleeplessness, or
from mind-wandering when they are engaged
on some task which requires concentration.
The attempt to get rid of such things as these
by mental methods is as reasonable and
sensible an aim as the attempt to get rid of
one's bodily weaknesses by the use of dumb-
bells. These are the kinds of mental defect
about which we do not go to see the doctor.
They are, however, a source of reduced
mental efficiency, and we have not yet got
a profession of " mental straighteners " (as
suggested by Samuel Butler in *Erewhon*) to
whom we can go to be treated for the minor
ailments of our minds just as we can go to a
doctor for a cold.

It may, therefore, be worth while to make
a short survey of the methods of mental
development which have been used at various
times, in order to see whether there is anything of practical usefulness for the ordinary
person which we can glean from them. We
shall not take it for granted that any sort
of mental gymnastics which have been tried
by exceptional people in various parts of
the world must necessarily be useful to ourselves. On the other hand, we shall not

14

make up our minds that any attempt at mental development is necessarily foolish for the ordinary person.

There seems no reason, on the face of it, why it should be more eccentric to use mental exercises for mental improvement than to use dumb-bell exercises for physical improvement. It is true, of course, that the use of dumb-bells can never really take the place in physical development of a free and healthy use of the muscles in hard out-door work. But dumb-bells are meant for the people who necessarily have an indoor occupation which makes it impossible for them to be developing their muscles in the original and natural out-door way. The same is true of the use of exercises for mental development. They can never be useful to those whose minds already work with perfect efficiency, and it would be absurd to suggest to the kind of brain-worker whose daily task makes him concentrate arduously all the time that he should do artificial mental exercises for concentration. His work will give him all the exercise in concentration that he needs. It is not, however, for such mental athletes that this book is written.

What scheme of mental development any

person carries out must, of course, depend on what ideal of mental attainment he considers a reasonable one. This question of aim is an important one, and we must spend a few minutes thinking about it. The difficulty does not occur in the same way with physical exercises. A man may, without doing himself much harm, spend ten minutes a day pushing dumb-bells about with no more definite idea than the vague one of developing his body. It is doubtful whether he could do anything useful at all in the way of developing his mind without a much clearer idea of what he was aiming at.

The Yogis taught a system of control by means of which a man could learn to think about nothing at all and could remain absolutely untouched by his affections and by the demands of outside things. The Stoics taught a more moderate discipline by which a man could be released from the bondage of his emotions so that he would be influenced by neither pity nor anger, though still (as in every other system) he was under the necessity of carrying out conduct for the good of his fellow men. No doubt, if we followed their methods we could become Yogis or Stoics, but do we want

16

to? If we do not, we can expect to get little profit from just dipping here and there into the exercises described by the Yogis and Stoics, and carrying them out without having any clear aim in view.

Some years ago, a little book was published entitled *How to be a Yogi*. Perhaps if we followed its instructions for a sufficient number of years, we should all be able to become Yogis. But it is reasonable to ask first " Do I want to become a Yogi? "

For myself, I am perfectly clear about the answer. I do not at all want to be a Yogi. I have no ambition to be able to think about nothing, and I do not want to be free from desire. It would be convenient to be able to free myself from those desires which I cannot fulfil, but I am not willing to purchase this freedom at the cost of losing my enjoyment of food and drink, of the mountains and sea, and of losing my power of loving other persons. The Yogi may tell me that these desires bring sorrow to the person possessing them. That I know, and I judge that they are worth it. I do not, therefore, want to be a Yogi, and the mental exercises which would make me into one are of no use to me.

Every system in the past has had some definite aim, although these aims have differed widely. I suppose few of us could unreservedly accept the aims of the Yogis or of the Buddhists. More would be willing to accept the aims of Ignatius Loyola. It seems to be a peculiarity of our own times that we have books recommending us to practise mental exercises without any clear object at all.

I once bought a book on concentration which contained a series of instructions, one of which was to hold the image of a chair in the mind for as long as possible without allowing it to waver. At this point, the ordinary person very properly asks " Why ? " and the author of the book gives him no answer. It is difficult to see why one should be better off through being able to think of a chair steadily for ten minutes or even for ten hours. Most of the thinking about chairs which any of us need to do in practice can be done quite effectively in ten seconds. What, then, is the object of this exercise ? It is true that there are similar exercises in the Yogi systems, but these form an essential link in the ideal of attaining isolation from the world. Most of us, however, would agree to reject this ideal.

The author may have known what was his object in this exercise, but certainly he did not explain it. Until he does, we may reasonably refuse to waste our time in concentrating on chairs. Exercises in concentration are, for many people, well worth carrying out, but it is more reasonable to practise concentration on some material worth while in itself—on some poem, for example, familiarity with which will be a permanent enrichment to the mind, or on the study of some branch of science, or even on the efficient performance of the task by which one earns one's living.

It should hardly be necessary to say that by mental methods one can only gain mental results. Physical results can only follow from physical means. Many writers and lecturers on this subject promise their followers wealth, perfect health, and beauty. But these are obviously external things which can only follow indirectly and in a very limited way from any process of mental development. Mental exercises may increase your desire for wealth and even your business efficiency, but if you are dependent for your livelihood on inadequate wages or on the interest from shares in a worked-out gold mine, no amount of mental exercising will save you from being poor. Similarly it is childish and unscientific to look to mental methods to cure you of an ulcerated stomach or a hare-lip.

Mental methods may give you contentment with your physical limitations, they cannot remove them. It is true that the illness which results from fears and unsatisfied desires (and, no doubt, a great deal of illness is of this kind), and the ugliness which results from harbouring ugly thoughts may be cured by suitable mental exercises producing thoughts of health, confidence and benevolence. That, however, is all. There still remain economic conditions, bacteria, and physical disfigurements which must be fought by other methods. It is mere dishonesty when the pseudo-psychological writer wins disciples by promising them unbounded wealth, health and beauty, by means which can never alone be sufficient to win them.

We now come to the really important practical question. If we have decided to reject the ideals of the Yogis, and even of the Stoics—all stern ascetics who would take away too much of the ordinary joy of living—what remains as a reasonable ideal for our mental development?

For the purpose of this book, I propose to take a very simple one—mental efficiency. Our minds are instruments with which we must work. We must be able to think accurately, to remember what is important and to forget what is trivial, to feel such emotions as will lead us to useful activities and to shut out those which are merely painful or useless; we must be able to sleep calmly at night as well as to think clearly by day; we must be able to judge correctly on disputed questions without being influenced by our prejudices or by unreasoning emotions, and we must have those dispositions of character which will lead us to conduct good in itself and serviceable to other people.

Perhaps I may be asked why I have chosen to take mental efficiency and not happiness as the goal to be aimed at in our mental development. Happiness may, at first sight, seem to be the obvious thing to pursue, but the wisdom of the past and the present unite in telling us that happiness is a quarry too elusive to be captured by direct pursuit.

There are two theories about the pursuit of happiness which are widely held. The first is the theory that the aim of all the activity of men is the winning of happiness; the second theory is that it ought to be. Sometimes both theories are upheld by the same people. These people believe that men, on the whole, do seek happiness and that they ought to, although they are often ignorant of the right way to find it.

I do not believe that either of these theories is true. Men seek other things than happiness, such as wealth or fame. They do not try to win these things because they think that they will bring them happiness, but because these seem to them to be ends attractive in themselves. Men may find more or less of happiness in the attainment of wealth, love or fame, or in the mere attempt to gain them, but it is a misunderstanding of human nature to suppose that men do not really want these things but only the happiness that they suppose will be the result of them. On the contrary, those who pursue such ends most ardently and most effectively will generally be found to be those who are least occupied with thoughts about happiness.

22

Indeed those who are always clamouring for happiness are not normal, but will generally be found to belong to the ranks of those ineffective people who have not satisfactorily adapted themselves to the demands of life. They are on a road which leads neither to happiness nor to efficiency. If a man is in pursuit of reasonable ends and pursues these in an efficient manner, he will be as happy as external circumstances and the peculiarities of his own disposition allow him to be. Mental efficiency may thus promote a man's happiness : the conscious pursuit of happiness will neither increase his mental efficiency nor, in the long run, his happiness.

This ideal of efficiency, if it is not so picturesque as the attainment of isolation by the destruction of desire, and not so seductive as the pursuit of happiness, will give us plenty to do.

Chapter II   Auto-suggestion—Its Uses and Limitations

A METHOD of mental control which recommends itself because of its simplicity and its usefulness is the one called " auto-suggestion " or " self-suggestion." This is the method in which one tries to produce some change in one's mind by saying to oneself a form of words—sending oneself to sleep by saying " I am falling asleep," or trying to keep oneself from sea-sickness by repeating " I am enjoying this voyage and I am feeling fit and well."

This method of mental control is, in fact, very often successful. Undoubtedly it is more successful with some people than with others, and it is more successful in some tasks than in others. We may find ourselves able to send ourselves to sleep by auto-suggestion when there is no reason for staying awake except that we are in unaccustomed surroundings. We may, on the other hand, be much less successful when we are lying awake worrying about some question of money, and quite unsuccessful if what is keeping us awake is a violent toothache. It may be worth while to mention at this point, that, if we do want to use auto-suggestion for sending ourselves to sleep when there is something like a worry or a pain which is keeping us awake, the best method is first to use a formula for the removal of the source of disturbance—one suggesting calmness or freedom from pain—and when that has been successful use the ordinary auto-suggestion for producing sleep.

One striking and quite useful thing for which the method of auto-suggestion may be employed is for waking ourselves up at a prescribed hour in the morning. If we wish to wake ourselves at some unusual time, it is sufficient to repeat to ourselves that we will wake up at that time, and we find that we do. Since waking up at a desired time cannot be done voluntarily in any more direct way, this is a very striking psychological experiment which should convince any sceptical person of the reality of auto-suggestion. Practically, however, I have found it open to two objections. First, if I rely on this method I find myself liable to wake earlier than the prescribed time (sometimes more than once); secondly, on rare occasions (particularly when I am very tired) the method fails. It is, therefore, generally better in practice to rely on an alarm clock.

The most useful field of auto-suggestion will be found to lie in those activities in which neither a convenient piece of mechanism such as an alarm clock nor our ordinary powers of willed activity help us. Such, for example, are : going to sleep, getting rid of the slight but annoying conditions of depression or irritability which affect all of us at times, removing annoying thoughts which will intrude when we wish to be busy with something else, or overcoming the fear which assails us when we have to speak in public or when we find ourselves at a great height above the ground.

In any case our method of using auto-suggestion will be to frame a suitable formula to repeat to ourselves. " I shall cease to be disturbed by this thought and will be able to apply myself to my work easily and with concentration " would, for example, be a suitable formula against an obsessing thought or worry. " I shall speak boldly and well "

29

would be a suitable auto-suggestion against the fear of an audience. It should be couched in the form of confident assertion— not " I must " or " I hope to," but " I shall." Yet it should not be so absolute as to arouse in our minds an inevitable contradiction. " I am falling asleep " is a reasonable auto-suggestion against wakefulness, but " I am asleep " would be a plain and unconvincing lie which would probably fail in its object.

Having decided on a formula suitable for the particular auto-suggestion we wish to make, the next thing is to repeat the formula many times over to ourselves (let us say twenty times or more). The repetition should be with the mouth. The formula should either be said audibly or sub-vocally (with the lips moving but without making any sound); it should not be merely thought. M. Coué recommends that the formula should be gabbled, but it is possible that individuals differ in this respect. Many people find it more effective to repeat the formula in a deliberate manner as we should if we were making a confident statement to someone else. I should recommend that the formula be repeated many times, with movement of the lips but without sound, and in a deliberate manner.

About the use of auto-suggestion for curing diseases, it is necessary to speak with a good deal of caution. Certain disease symptoms may be produced by the mind alone. These may range from simple headaches to conditions which to all outward appearance seem to be cases of serious bodily trouble such as kidney disease or rheumatoid arthritis. Of course, the person who produces all the symptoms of kidney disease, although his kidneys themselves are really in perfect working order, is not a mentally well person. He (or more probably she) is a victim of the mental disease of hysteria, which can simulate the symptoms of a large variety of physical disorders.

Since these symptoms have no real existence but are produced by the mind of the person suffering from them, it is reasonable to hope that they may be cured by mental means. But there are also genuine physical disorders which are not mentally caused and cannot be mentally cured. Because we read of cases of apparent paralytics cured by auto-suggestion under the influence of that talented exponent of auto-suggestion,

M. Coué, we must not jump to the con-
clusions that a true paralytic whose condition has been caused by the destruction
of a trunk motor-nerve through injury or
disease could have been similarly cured. It
is quite certain that he could not.

No doubt there is a factor in the recovery
from even physical diseases which is affected
by our minds. We are more likely to recover
from an illness if we feel confident of recovery,
and in any case the bodily healing process
itself may be aided by auto-suggestion.
Auto-suggestions of confidence and returning
health may profitably be used, but we must
not rely on auto-suggestion for physical
troubles when physical methods are necessary. We may use auto-suggestion to give
us a confident attitude of mind and to assist
the natural processes of healing even when
we are suffering from a broken leg, but we
must not allow our faith in auto-suggestion
to make us neglect the services of a surgeon
to set the leg. If we do, the results will be
disastrous.

There are two dangers in the use of auto-
suggestion for the cure of disease. First,
there is the possibility that the habit of
relying on auto-suggestion may be a danger-

ous one for the very persons who are prone to these " diseases of the imagination." One thing that is the matter with them is that their bodies too easily act out suggestions of illness received from their minds. When they try to cure themselves by auto-suggestion, they are accustoming their bodies still further to act out suggestions received in this mechanical way from their minds. In other words, they are strengthening by practice the very tendency which produced their illness.   What they really need is often a mental discipline for strengthening their power of willed control, rather than a removal of their particular symptoms by auto-suggestion.

The second danger is that auto-suggestion may remove symptoms without removing their underlying physical causes.   If a man suffers from toothache, he may succeed in removing the pain of it by auto-suggestion. But if he really has a decaying tooth, suggesting away the pain will not stop the tooth from decaying and it may make him neglect to go to the dentist.   If he does not go to the dentist, he is no more sensible than the man in the ever-recurring joke about auto-suggestion who sits by his broken-down motor-car and repeats the formula : " **My car** is working better and better." He **is** making the mistake of relying on mental methods to produce physical results.

Most of us, however, are sensible people and will not be guilty of such imbecilities. We will rely on mental methods only for the production of mental results, and we may use auto-suggestion in our illnesses with discretion and profit, not allowing it to take the place of physical methods when these are necessary. We may save ourselves from a sleepless night by auto-suggesting away the pain of toothache, but we will also resolve to visit the dentist the next day. Similarly we may use auto-suggestion to get rid of worrying thoughts about money which **are** disturbing our night's rest, but we will **also** resolve to reduce our expenditure until it is less than our income. Used in this **way**, auto-suggestion will be a useful mental medicine. Used in the other way it may **be** a dangerous drug.

There is another limitation of the use of auto-suggestion to which it is necessary **to** draw attention. This is that the method of auto-suggestion should not be used to take the place of the direct control of our actions and thoughts which we call " willing." Willing is something so much more commonplace and familiar than auto-suggestion that we are likely to forget it when we are talking about methods of mental control. Yet the development of the power of willed control over our bodily and mental activities must not be forgotten in a scheme of mental development. In exploring the unusual methods of exercising mental control, we must not forget the commonplace ones.

The things that happen in ourselves—in our minds and bodies—are of three kinds. Some are automatic, such as the beating of our heart, the forgetting of the things that have happened to us in the past, and the healing of a bodily or mental wound. These are called " automatic " because they go on by themselves and we cannot in any direct way either help them or stop them. Opposite to these automatic activities are such things as striking a match, getting out of bed, or solving a puzzle. These are " willed " activities. Lastly, there is the kind of mental or bodily happening which is in between those two. These are happenings which are partly automatic but partly under our control. The action of breathing is a familiar example. Our bodily and mental habits are important members of this class. Such things as the actions of shaving or the processes of thought and feeling which go on when we think along some familiar line (let us say, on politics) are mainly automatic, but we can attend to them by an effort of attention and control them if we want to.

A recent exponent of a system of mental control has put forward the aim that we should make all bodily habits into willed actions—that we should be fully conscious of and should have complete control of the movements made, for example, in sitting down in a chair. It is difficult to see what gain there would be in this. Our minds allow such movements to drop out of consciousness and to become automatic so that our conscious attention may be occupied with more important things. It is a general rule that processes of body which would not profit by our willed interference become automatic. It would be of no benefit to us to be able to control the beating of our hearts, and it would be a waste of time to try, although it is quite possible that we could learn to do it if we tried hard enough. When our automatic bodily processes are going on quite well by themselves they are best left alone.

Now it is obvious that a great part of the working of our minds is similarly automatic. The general attitudes of our mind towards persons and things and towards its own processes and towards the processes of its body are all automatic—they go on by themselves without our conscious interference.

What we are trying to do in auto-suggestion is to get some control over those processes of our minds which commonly go on by themselves. It may be objected that we ought not to use auto-suggestion because it is best to leave the automatic actions of our mind to take care of themselves so long as they are working satisfactorily. There is much good sense in this objection. So long as the automatic activities of our minds are going on satisfactorily it is unwise to interfere with them by auto-suggestion or by any other method. Medicine should only be used when we are sick and not when our bodies are working properly. Auto-suggestion is a medicine of the mind and not a food.

I have just said that we can leave the

automatic activities of our minds to take care of themselves *so long as they are going on satisfactorily.* It is necessary to emphasise that condition. If we are lying awake in bed at night, if our minds are haunted by a worrying thought, or if we find ourselves unable to concentrate on a task which demands concentrated attention, then the automatic activities of our minds are not working to our satisfaction. If we cannot put right what is wrong by direct willing, then we shall be wise to use the method of auto-suggestion.

Let us be clear what is meant by " willing." It is something perfectly obvious and commonplace. If I move a finger because I choose to, or if I get up and walk to the door, or if I decide to start thinking about my summer holiday, these are all " willed " activities. They are things which would not have taken place if I had decided against them.

There is, however, another and wrong sense in which the word " willing " is used. I have an occult book which gives as an exercise for developing the " astral body " that one should sit in a chair and, with eyes closed, " will " oneself to be out of it. What the author means is that one should think intensely of oneself as out of the chair. But this is not willing, it is merely a particular kind of wishing. If you sit in a chair and really will to get up, you get up. This is the evidence that you have willed to get up. You could only go on sitting in a chair and " willing " to be out if you were tied there, and even then you would make all the movements of straining against the ropes in your attempt to get up. Sitting in a chair and thinking strenuously of getting up without sending the necessary nervous impulses from the brain to the limbs whose movements would get you up is the most fatuous substitute for willing that can well be imagined. This is an obviously wrong use of the word " will." The sign that you " will " something is that you do it (unless forcibly prevented).

We have already seen that certain automatic happenings of our minds and bodies cannot be brought directly under our power of willing. There are a great many others, however, which can. Examples are such activities as walking, talking, thinking and remembering. Auto-suggestion should not be used for directing these willed activities.

39

For example, if we want to get out of bed on a cold morning, the right way to do it is to make a strenuous willed effort which gets us up, not to repeat to ourselves the formula : " I am just going to get out of bed." This is a part of our behaviour over which we have direct control and it is important not to lose this power of willed control. It is impossible to estimate the gain to us which results from the fact that we have a direct kind of control over our thinking and talking which we have not over our sleeping and the beating of our heart.

The power of willed control over thoughts and actions is a power of the mind which is, at least, as well worth cultivation and development as any other. The person who can do things simply because he chooses to do them (such as standing his ground when he is afraid, or stopping smoking when he wants to) has a more efficient mental apparatus than the person who can not. How are we to cultivate this power of willing? Like most other things it improves with practice and is weakened by neglect. It must be cultivated by constant exercise. William James recommended that we should all practise our power of willing by doing something we do not want to do every day simply for the sake of developing this side of our characters. Many persons, of course, have to do every day many things they strongly dislike. Such persons may face these necessary evils boldly and so develop their power of willing. Those, however, who lead easy lives may often have to make their opportunities for strenuous efforts of this kind.

Where we have this power of willed control over our bodily or mental processes, it should be developed and we should make no attempt to supplement it by the use of auto-suggestion. Auto-suggestion steps in as a method for gaining control over those processes which are automatic and therefore out of our direct control. For this purpose we shall find it a useful instrument.

Chapter III   How Habits may be Formed and Broken

IF I move my arm or one of my fingers in a new way, it is easier for me to make that same movement again. This is the first law of bodily habit. It states the well-known fact that movements improve and become easier by practice. Also we know that a new action is, at first, clearly present to our consciousness, and it is more under our control than it will ever be again. If we go on making this same movement, it becomes more and more automatic. It seems to go on by itself, and little effort is needed on our part. Instead we may find that an effort is required to stop ourselves from making the movement. The first carrying out of a new bodily or mental activity prepares, as it were, a track for its future happening so that it takes place more easily and more inevitably.

The final stage in this development is when actions constantly repeated seem to take care of themselves, and checking them by willed effort has become difficult or impossible.

They have then become *automatic*. If the activity is one which we want to carry out (such as the movements in a game), we say that we have acquired skill in it. If it is one that we do not want to carry out, we say that we have contracted a bad habit.

The same is true of mental habits. If I think a thought once, that thought more easily comes back. The more often I feel an emotion, the more easily will that emotion occur again. After a time, it may require an effort to stop myself from thinking a familiar thought in a familiar way. The stage in thought-habits corresponding to the automatic stage in bodily habits is when they become obvious, when they seem to think themselves and it seems impossible to doubt them. Such obvious habitual thoughts are, for example, that only one straight line can be drawn between two points, that our political opponents are stupid or wicked, and that two and two make four. Many other thoughts, even judgments about persons and things, have acquired this obviousness through habitual use. Yet these apparently obvious and certain judgments must very often be false, because the habitual

46

judgments of one man may be quite different from those of his neighbour. We cannot all be right about the things we feel certain of.

There is another law of bodily habit. If I repeat two movements together, or one after the other, then, whenever I afterwards perform one movement, the other is strongly inclined to accompany it or to follow it. In this way, we form groups or chains of habitual bodily movements. Such are to be found in shaving or in the complicated set of movements used in making a stroke in a game of skill. If we go on repeating them these groups of movements too become finally automatic. The movements made, for example, in opening a door become so familiar to us that we need only push our hand towards a door-knob and the rest of the necessary movements carry themselves out without our intervention and without our having any consciousness of them.

This again is also true of mental habits. Two or more thoughts or feelings which have occurred together more than once tend to occur together again. The laws by which they are grouped together are called the Laws of Mental Association. They are really laws of the formation of mental habits. For example, if a child has frequently had the feeling of fear when he has seen a dog, the feeling of fear will be more and more strongly and finally perhaps inevitably called up by the sight of a dog. If a man has heard violent language and has felt angry feelings many times in connection with the members of a particular political party with which he does not agree, he finally forms a habit of thinking such violent thoughts and feeling angry emotions whenever he meets or thinks of members of this party. He has formed a mental habit of which he has more or less completely lost control. If, as is probable, the reproaches are unjust and the anger is unnecessary he has formed a mental habit which is thoroughly unserviceable. Such unserviceable mental habits are what we ordinarily call " unreasonable prejudices." This habit prevents its possessor from acting reasonably and from thinking calmly about a certain group of questions.

Unhappily, the man himself is probably not discontented with such emotional and intellectual habits. Many people (and even highly intelligent people) wear their social and political prejudices with as much satisfaction as if they were a row of medals.

Their satisfaction, however, does not alter the fact that these habits interfere with the usefulness of their mental processes. No scheme of mental control would, therefore, be adequate which did not attempt to remove such prejudices and to replace them by more serviceable habits of thought.

This tendency of our actions and thoughts to become more and more mechanical and so to elude our control seems to many people to be a depressing fact. Even William James suggests that in most of us, by the age of thirty, the character has set like plaster, and will never soften again. We seem to be like trams which lay their own tracks in the first place but which afterwards go on running in them with only occasional variations.

Some people are so depressed by this prospect that they are willing to adopt as a principle in their lives the attempt to break all the chains of their habits. Yet not all habit formation is objectionable. Much of it is essential in any efficient and well-ordered life. It is through the familiar everyday things such as shaving, sitting down, and mentally digesting the morning's news becoming automatic through habit, that we have energy and attention to devote to other

D   49

things. No man could develop a business or write a book or engage in any other activity requiring new action and new thought, if he still had to give to shaving or to writing his name the concentrated attention that was necessary when these were new actions. By having made these into habits he has time and energy to spare for other things.

For this reason, William James advised his readers to make all the details of their daily lives into habits, in order to avoid the waste of effort which results from having to think about them. Opposite to this is the practice of a recent teacher of mental control who is reported to have made a principle of breaking down all the pre-formed habits of his disciples, their times of eating, of going to bed, and so on.

Although these seem to be opposite ideals, a little reflection will show that there is a certain amount of sense in both. Ordinarily such things as eating, sleeping, etc., must be habits, but it is a great gain if we can at will break across these rigid ordinary habits of action and thought so that we can release ourselves from slavery to them. Then we shall be able to choose freely whether we are to retain them for the future or to form new ones.

50

This breaking across our ordinary habits is perhaps one of the mental advantages we gain from such a holiday as one in which we camp out, thus interfering with all our ordinary habits of eating, sleeping, sitting down, and so on. Even if such systematic interference with ordinary habits were made a feature of the discipline we imposed on ourselves in a course of mental control, it clearly could not be with the object of permanently freeing ourselves from all habits. As we have already seen, this would cause a tremendous waste of time and energy. The only reasonable aim in such a wholesale destruction of old habits is an attempt to get the mastery of them so that we can be free to choose which of them we are going to keep and which we are going to replace by new habits.

It is of no use simply to regret this tendency of our bodies, of our nervous systems, and of our minds, to form habits. We must accept it and make use of it. If this peculiarity of our bodily and mental make-up makes it more difficult for us to break off a bad habit, it also makes it easier for us to form a good one. If it is true that every time we (let us say) use bad language, it becomes easier for us to use bad language again, it is

51

also true that every time we control our tendency to use bad language by willed effort, it is easier to control it again. What it amounts to is that we must attempt to form the habits we want to form by repetition, and we must break the habits we want to break by never allowing them a repetition. We cannot choose to have no habits at all, but we can choose what habits we shall have. We must use the fact of habit formation as an ally in our attempt to gain mental control and not always treat it as an enemy.

The method of breaking a habit is simply by refusing, by willed effort, to allow it any repetition. Simple as this sounds, it may, of course, be a task of almost insuperable difficulty. There is no easy way of overcoming a deeply-rooted habit, although there are methods of lightening the difficulty. Suitable auto-suggestions may sometimes be used successfully to reduce the strength of the craving to return to a habit we have decided to abandon. Another way of making the process less hard is always to perform some other action when one feels the impulse to carry out the old habit. A simple example of this is, when trying to break oneself of smoking cigarettes, to put a small hard sweet into one's mouth whenever one feels the craving to light a cigarette. In the same way, a student, let us say, struggling against a persistent habit may find that if he deliberately applies himself to his work every time he feels the impulse to his habit, the difficulty of resisting it will grow less and finally disappear.

When it is not a question of a simple bodily habit but of the much more complex situation of a drug habit, the difficulty may be very great. In attempting to cure a habit of drug-taking, it is not simply a habit of a few muscles that has to be broken, but one formed by the whole body and mind, a habit of the nervous system, of the digestive system, and so on. If the supply of drug is stopped, a physiological craving is set up which no effort of the mind can stop from being acutely painful even though willed effort may be successful in resisting its impulse.

In all cases of breaking a habit, the ideal is to permit no exception at all to the rule of not carrying out the habitual action in question, once the fight against it has started. This ideal rule cannot always be carried out strictly. In breaking the addiction to some kinds of drug, for example, the bodily and mental disturbance which would result from a sudden stoppage of the drug may be so severe as to be dangerous. In these cases, the dose must be decreased gradually. The ideal rule of complete and absolute stoppage of the offending habit should, however, always be followed when it is possible.

Habits of thought and feeling also demand our attention. We form habits of always feeling anger at the mention of some persons or of the members of some nations; and we also form habits of feeling fear in some situations (as when children feel fear in the dark, some psycho-neurotic persons feel fear in all enclosed places, and most of us feel fear on heights). These are habits of feeling. Similarly there are habits of thought and speech, which determine what we shall believe and say about certain questions. The fact that we embrace a political or religious creed means that we have accepted certain habits of thought, so that on a certain number of new questions our minds are, in effect, already made up. When a line of thought becomes thoroughly habitual it appears to us to be self-evident or obvious, and we are surprised that it does not appear to be so to other people, and we suspect them of being biassed and unreasonable. Yet the fact that a line of thought appears obvious may mean nothing except that we have thought it so often that it has become a mental habit. It is no guarantee that the thought is true.

Of course, mental habits, like bodily ones, have their use. They make us consistent. That, in itself, is a great gain practically. If we had no thought habits, our judgments would vary from day to day, and we might find ourselves on the platform of a prohibitionist league on one night and on the platform of a society supporting the liquor trade the next night. That would be a great inconvenience.

Also thought habits effect a great saving of mental energy. It is because we do not have to make up our minds afresh on every question that presents itself, that we have time and energy to spare for careful thought on other questions. A scientist would have little time or energy for thinking about the atomic theory if he had not made up his mind on thousands of other questions, such as the relative merits of Turkish and Virginian cigarettes, the prohibition question,

55

and the programmes of the three political parties.

The disadvantage of thought habits is that while they give us consistency and save us trouble, they may prevent us from acquiring new truth. Indeed, the breaking of old habits of thought is generally a condition which we have to fulfil in order to get nearer to the truth. The habit of thinking that the sun went round the earth was so deeply ingrained in men that it seemed to them to be an obvious truth which one would be a fool to deny until Copernicus shook himself free from this thought habit and showed that it was the earth which moved round the sun.

To come nearer to our own times, a lot of statements about space and time seemed obvious even to those who had thought most carefully about the subject (such as that the length of a rigid rod was always the same and could not be affected by the movement of the rod) until Einstein showed that nothing but long mental habit made these things appear obvious, for they were not exactly true. The difference, of course, was small enough not to be noticeable under ordinary conditions of observation. That was why we had formed the habit. But physicists were beginning to study conditions under which the difference was important and were unable to make new conquests of scientific truth until Einstein had liberated them from their old habits of thought.

"To think accurately" was one of the aims we admitted as part of that state of mental efficiency which we agreed to regard as the aim of mental control. Thinking accurately must often mean an attempt to break down the obvious judgments which spring from thought habits. The habit of suspecting that our easiest judgments may rest on nothing more profound than our habits of thought should be one of the results of anything that can fairly be called a "liberal education."

One way in which this habit can be acquired is by consistently reading newspapers and books putting forward views with which we disagree. This might well be a piece of mental discipline for everyone desirous of keeping his mental processes under control. Mere unsympathetic reading with ejaculations of "nonsense," "rubbish," at every unwelcome suggestion will be useless. Our thought habits will not even begin to be broken down until we can read such papers and books with sympathetic understanding, really entering into the new and unfamiliar thought of our opponent. Then we shall have started on the path of making a free choice in our opinions, and escaping from bondage to our old habits of thought.

In all attempts to overcome habits— habits of thought, of feeling, and of action —we must remember that it cannot be a reasonable aim to get rid of all habits. That would be to produce a condition of mind of hopeless inefficiency—a condition which we might describe as " mental anarchy." Our aim must be the more moderate but very important one of being able to choose freely which of our habits we are going to keep and which we are going to abandon.

I<small>F</small>, for the sake of a psychological experiment, you approach a gentleman sitting quietly in a tram and pull his beard, tweak his nose or call him a fool, you may notice that your experiment is followed by several interesting physiological and psychological changes. The rate of your subject's heartbeat will increase and the distension of the small veins in his skin will cause him to flush. The frontal muscles will pull down his eyebrows, causing the lines to appear between them which we call a frown. If you watch his upper lip closely you may notice a slight tendency of the corners of his mouth to rise. This is a relic of the snarl of the animals which attack with their powerful canine teeth. You may also notice a tendency of the hair at the back of the gentleman's head to raise itself and stand on end.

The most important bodily change, however (which may make the exact examination of these other changes difficult), will be the impulse to violent behaviour. The subject of your experiment will either strike you, or at least will experience an impulse to strike, which is likely to be shown by a clenching of his fists. The striking, itself, may have its place taken by the use of violent and abusive language. At the same time, if you question your subject, you will find that he is experiencing an unpleasant feeling of peculiar quality which he will call " feeling angry." The whole condition to which you have reduced the gentleman is an example of a condition known as an emotion. It is the emotion of anger.

Another set of bodily and mental changes takes place when a man is strolling in a field and notices a bull approaching him in a threatening manner. The condition which the bull will produce under these circumstances is the emotion of fear.

A person under the influence of strong emotion tends to behave violently and in a manner which seems to show clearly to the onlookers that his body is, to some extent, like a machine out of control. While he behaves violently, such a man is unable to think clearly. This loss of clearness in thinking may even make his behaviour less effective than it would have been if he were not under the influence of strong emotion. A boxer does not box best when he is angry. A really angry man may be less capable of making effective, stinging remarks to his opponent than if he had controlled his anger. Although fear makes it possible for one to run faster and harder than would have been possible in a normal condition, the uncontrolled and unreasoning way in which the frightened person runs may actually prevent his escape from danger.

The behaviour which results from strong emotion shows, then, a somewhat mechanical character. The man who is very much angry or afraid is rather like a motor-car over which the driver has no control. The emotions are, in fact, due to a very mechanical part of our nervous system. They are not results of the activity of the brain, which is the part of our nervous system that thinks and reflects and controls. They are not even started by the part of the nervous system to which the brain belongs. Emotions result from the action of a very primitive part of our nervous system called the autonomic nervous system. This is the system of which the solar plexus is a part and which works in co-operation with certain of the glands, such as the thyroid gland.

It is because of this mechanical nature of the emotions that systems of mental culture have always had as part of their aim the control of emotions. Plato and Buddha, the Stoics and the exponents of New Thought, are all alike in trying to teach people ways of subjugating their emotions, although they have differed a good deal in how far they have wanted to destroy the emotions altogether. It appeared to these thinkers that a man acting under strong emotion was less of a man and more of a machine or a beast. Even if we confine ourselves to the simple aim of mental efficiency, we cannot be content to leave our emotions unregulated. Highly emotional behaviour is very generally highly inefficient behaviour.

There is an obvious difficulty in the control of the emotions which must strike us at once. There is an essential part of the emotions which is not under willed control at all. We cannot control the beating of our heart, or the blood supply to our skin, by any willed effort however great. At the same time, it seems certain that if these changes of our skin and blood take place we shall feel emotion. If, for example, when we see a bull, the blood is driven from our skin, our heart beats faster, and our knees start trembling, then we shall feel fear. If the emotion of fear follows from something that we cannot control, in what possible manner can we control our fear?

The answer to this question takes us to the root of the psychological problem of controlling the emotions. It is perfectly true that there is a part of the emotion which we cannot directly control. It is also true, however, that there is a part we can control. This part is the bodily behaviour and the facial expression to which the emotion gives rise. While the frightened man cannot stop himself from turning pale, he can stop himself by willed effort from running away or from showing the expression of the emotion of fear in his face. Of course, in any particular case of fear, the impulse to run away and to show fear by the movements of the face may be so strong that the effort required to control them is greater than the person in question is capable of. They are, however, theoretically still controllable, and how far a man is actually able to control them depends not only on how strong they are, but also on how far he has developed his capacity for willed effort. If he wants to master his fear, it is these controllable bodily changes that he will attack and, as he successfully controls them, both the involuntary bodily changes (such as the turning pale) and the unpleasant feeling itself will tend to disappear.

We may perform some simple experiments which will show us the influence of our bodily behaviour and expressions of face on our feelings. If you try drawing your eyebrows down in a frown and clenching your fists, you will begin to feel yourself experiencing an emotion of anger even although there is nothing to be angry about. If, on the other hand, when you have something to be angry about you make an effort to keep your forehead smooth and your hands open, the feeling of anger will grow less and will rapidly disappear altogether. In the same way, if you sit in a chair with your muscles relaxed, your head bowed down and your mouth drooping you will begin to feel depressed. If, when you are depressed about something, you brace up the muscles of your back, making your body erect, and pull your mouth into a smile you will find that the depression fades away.

The first principle, then, in the control of the emotions is this. While the feeling part of your emotion is not itself under willed control, the facial expression and the behaviour of the emotion can be controlled more or less. Whether less or more depends partly on the violence of the emotion at the moment, but partly also on the extent to which you have habitually practised control of these things. You cannot stop yourself by a direct effort from feeling afraid when, let us say, you get up for the first time to address an audience, but you can stop yourself from looking cowed and from running away, and success in overcoming these controllable parts of the emotion will tend to result in the feeling itself disappearing too.

Another useful principle in the control of the emotions is that reflective thought about the object causing emotion tends to make the emotion disappear. This was a principle which was well understood by the Roman Stoics and by the Buddhists. The Stoic Emperor Marcus Aurelius Antoninus reminded his readers that the expensive wine they sought after was nothing but moisture squeezed from a grape, and that the rich purple robes which filled them with pride were nothing but sheep's hair twisted together and stained with the blood of a kind of periwinkle. The Buddhists were taught to go into graveyards and to reflect on the changes which the bodies underwent so that they might cease to desire the pleasures of a life which was nothing but a series of changes in similar bodies. An exactly similar idea lies behind the reflection, when some occurrence rouses an undesirable emotion, that " it will make no difference a hundred years hence." These are all examples of emotion being dissipated by reflection about the nature of the objects calling out emotion.

A very similar principle is to be found in the teaching of Jesus to his disciples that they should abolish worry from their minds by considering (that is, reflecting on) the birds and the flowers which were taken care of and clothed by God without any anxious care on their part.

A knowledge of psychology ought to provide us with an abundance of reflections to prevent us from being carried away with anger at the behaviour of another person. We can not only consider the nature of his impulses and feelings, but we can also reflect on the physiological character of our own emotions. If the old gentleman with whom this chapter started had been a Stoic with some knowledge of modern psychology, he might have reflected in some such way as the following : " This young man who has just pulled my beard has done it under the influence of his instinct of curiosity. The result of his action has merely been a momentary tension of the hairs on my chin which has caused me only very slight and transitory discomfort and has had no other results either bad or good. Moreover, this emotion of anger which I feel is nothing but the echo in consciousness of a change in the blood supply to my skin and internal organs, and why should I, a free man, have my conduct dictated to me by the condition of my viscera ? " Long before he got to the end of these reflections he would find there was little left of the powerful emotion of anger with which he had started.

Whatever method of subjugating undesirable emotions we put forward, we must be prepared to face one objection. This is the objection of the man who says that reflective thinking and the willed control of behaviour and expression are all very well for slight emotions, but they are powerless in the face of great ones. Our advice may be good enough to save a man from painful worry when he has lost sixpence, but it is a useless remedy to offer him when he has lost the accumulated savings of his lifetime.

This is a real difficulty, although it is by no means fatal to the principles which have been suggested. It is true that no method of mental control can be used for the first time by a person while suffering under a great grief or while he is in terror or in a rage. The intensity of the emotion itself will effectually prevent him from either thinking calmly or controlling his muscles.

The practical conclusion to be drawn from this fact is that it is useless to wait until one is suffering from a very powerful emotion before beginning the practice of controlling emotions. One might as well start heavy weight lifting by starting at once on the heaviest weights without first having strengthened one's muscles on the lighter ones. The person who habitually controls his slighter emotional disturbances will find that he has developed the power to deal with his greater ones. It is the person who habitually gives way to painful worry over the loss of sixpence who is utterly overwhelmed by a more serious loss.

70

If we wish to be able to resist the painful and unserviceable emotions of grief, anger and fear, in serious crises, we should use all methods of control to resist them when they come in milder forms. We should, for example, make the habit of not worrying over a small loss of money or when we miss a train, of not allowing ourselves to give way to irritation when someone jostles us in a crowd, or to fear when a vehicle in which we are travelling narrowly escapes an accident. A distinguished general of conspicuous courage has confessed that he was led into the military career by the fact that he was so unusually timid that he was forced to be always practising the control of his fear until this control became a strong habit.

Our aim, however, cannot be to get rid of all emotions, for some emotions are desirable. The world would be much worse, for example, if all mothers and all lovers used psychological methods to get rid of their feelings of affection. The total destruction of all emotion has, as a matter of fact, sometimes been taught in the past as an aim, and other writers have taught the less extreme doctrine that all emotions should be moderate in amount.

71

Nor can we be content only with getting rid of undesirable emotions. This must be part of our aim; we must absolutely abolish from our lives all worry, all needless fears and anger against other persons. But this is not all. Other emotions are generally desirable. Such are, for example, pity and the sympathetic emotions generally, anger at evil things (such as disease, injustice and war) and the fear of what is really dangerous.

The methods we have described might, of course, be used to get rid of these desirable emotions as well, but the result would be to make our characters poorer and really less efficient. The light-minded person who manages not to be moved by sympathy or by indignation at real evils has a character we shall not wish to set up as an ideal.

The desirable emotions (or the habit of feeling emotions in situations in which they are desirable) can, in fact, be developed by the use of the same principle of cultivation by exercise as has already been described for the formation of good habits. They can also be cultivated by thought. Some parts of systems of meditation (such as those used by many religions) are attempts to use exercises of thought in order to cultivate desirable emotional habits. We may, for example, cultivate the habit of feeling the sorrows of other persons as if they were our own, by making ourselves think of their sorrows until we feel the pain of them in ourselves. Or we may hold the picture of someone who has injured us in our mind, and force ourselves to think kindly of him.

I see no reason for doubting that meditation consistently carried out for long periods of time is a powerful method for attaching emotion to new objects, or for detaching it from other objects. Let us suppose that someone carries out Ignatius Loyola's meditation on Hell in accordance with its author's instruction, using all kinds of mental imagery to picture its horrors to himself, not allowing his efforts to stop until the end of an hour, and repeating the meditation the prescribed number of times. It seems reasonably certain that he will have in the end a much increased fear of hell.

To most of us the end attained does not seem a desirable one, but might the method not have been used for ends which the most modern mind would recognise as desirable? There are, of course, other meditations in Loyola's system with whose objects we should

73

all sympathise. Apart, however, from religious objects altogether, there are ends which might well be served by systematic meditation. The effectiveness with which we judge and act in many matters is impaired by the little emotion that is called out by important things remote from our experience and by the unduly great emotion called out by unimportant things closely affecting ourselves.

The modern man or woman's book of meditations might include an exercise of an hour each morning picturing the discomforts of life in a tenement. Imagery of sight and smell might call up the smoky chimney and the week's washing airing in the room in which supper is served, the husband too tired by his day's work and too dulled by its monotony to be kind; the bodily feelings might be pictured of the woman who had the full burden of the crowded and muddled home up to a few days before the birth of her baby, and so on. Another exercise might be one in which we meditated on our bank-balances as the Buddhists meditated on their bodies, until our emotional detachment from our possessions was so complete that we could judge with even and unbiassed minds the desirability of legislation which would increase the income tax or of municipal action which would increase the rates.

Another reason why we cannot be content merely to try to get rid of all emotion is the fact that emotion is the great driving force to action. To abolish emotion would be like abolishing the steam from an engine. Without some degree of fear, we should not be sufficiently careful to avoid really dangerous things; without pity, we should not be sufficiently active in relieving distress; and without some measure of anger, we should not be sufficiently strenuous in fighting against evils. Our aim must be to be able to choose freely by what emotions we shall be influenced and what ones we shall reject. No emotions are, of course, desirable in all circumstances. The desirability of an emotion in any particular case, depends largely on the conduct it leads to. It is as important that a child should be taught to be afraid of a savage dog and of influenza germs, as that it should be taught not to be afraid of the dark.

Another point to be remembered is that while emotions may be serviceable to action they are always a hindrance to clear thinking.

We do not think clearly, logically and accurately when we are thinking in a state of anger or even when we are thinking in a state of tenderness. The reason why we make errors in our thinking is not, as the older philosophers used to suppose, because we are ignorant of the laws of logic, but because we think under the influence of emotion. I look forward to the day when it will be an offence punishable by a long term of imprisonment for a man to make a speech calling up strong emotions in people who have to make responsible decisions for which clear thought is necessary. I am thinking, for example, of such times as an election. The term of imprisonment would be no shorter for the sentimentalist who made his audience weep than for the master of invective who made them angry. Either should be imprisoned on a charge of having confused the thought processes of the electorate by inducing emotion.

If we wish to think correctly we must think, so far as we can, without emotion of any kind. When we have come to our decisions we can, of course, put all the emotion at our command into our subsequent actions. Calm thought must be the condition under which we select the emotional impulses which shall drive us to action. Our ideal must be to think calmly and to act emotionally.

This does not mean, of course, that the orator has no useful social function. His task should be that of inducing emotion when action and not calm judgment are needed. This would be the opposite of our present unreasonable arrangement. Now, when we have to make responsible decisions on the rival merits of Free Trade and Protection or of privately owned and nationalised industries, instead of having a calm presentation of the observations, statistics, etc., from which alone a correct conclusion can be drawn, we hear fiery addresses calculated to activate our emotions and to make impossible a rational decision on the problems. When, on the other hand, it is necessary for us to be stirred into action about some admitted evil, like the prevalence of smoke in our large towns, we are given a closely reasoned address by a gentle, spectacled professor who illustrates his remarks by lantern slides showing figures and graphs. This would be the ideal form for an election address, just as our present election addresses would be the ideal form for orations on smoke, sewage, microbes, or housing.

We must notice, too, how at the present time other methods of inducing emotion than oratory are also used often for the wrong ends. A kind of music, for example, which produces emotion and heightens activity is used by armies and to produce warlike emotions amongst civilians. War is not merely a useless but a highly undesirable way for civilised people to dissipate their energies, and if they have wars at all they should participate in them under conditions which allow them to realise to the full their sadness and futility.

There are, on the other hand, highly desirable activities, colourless and distasteful in themselves, which need the stimulation of martial music if they are to be carried out with enthusiasm. The day must come when dustmen and sanitary workers are led to their noble work by the music of the pipes and drums, and when they will point proudly to the medals on their breasts which were struck in commemoration of notable victories over dirt and disease.

WE cannot go far in the task of trying to regulate our emotions without discovering that we are up against a stiffer difficulty than we expected. Emotional behaviour checked in one direction has a trick of finding expression in some other direction. We may, for example, have successfully formed the habit of not giving way to violent behaviour or even to violent or reproachful language, and then find that we have formed a new habit of criticising and discussing the faults of our neighbours.

We may do this with the best (even with the most pious) intentions, but still it is criticising and fault-finding. In a moment of self-illumination, we may suddenly realise that the old tendency to hostile behaviour which belongs to the emotion of anger is coming out in a new direction.

It is rather as if we had discovered a persistent weed in the garden, and had just cut down the part of it which we could see above the ground and had neglected the long tap-root running below the surface, and the result had been simply that the weed had sprouted again from a new point on the root. Or, it is as if we had noticed steam escaping from a leak in a boiler, and after carefully stopping up the leak had discovered that the result of our care was simply that the pressure of steam had increased until it had forced itself out at a new leak at another point.

The trouble has been that the emotion itself was only a surface effect of something lying deeper in our character. This something is a permanent, deep-rooted disposition to feel and behave in the ways belonging to the emotion—a disposition which is inborn, which is the result of the way our bodies and nervous systems are made up, and which is inherited from a long line of ancestors human and pre-human. This inherited disposition is what we call an " instinct."

Instincts are generally named after the kind of behaviour they produce. We speak of " the instinct of pugnacity " which gives rise to the emotion of anger and to violent or pugnacious behaviour, of the " instinct of flight " which gives rise to the emotion of fear and to the behaviour of running away from danger, and the " sex-instinct " which gives rise to courting, mating and home-making, and to the emotion of tenderness or love.

The relationship of any emotion to its instinct is very like that of the weed to its tap-root or of the leak to the pressure of steam in the boiler. Cut off the head of the weed and not only will its tap-root not be killed, it will even be stimulated to increased activity. Stop up the leak in the boiler, and if the steam cannot find an outlet somewhere else it will blow up your boiler. In the same way, if you cut off all the obvious outlets of anger, your instinct of pugnacity may find new outlets in talking scandal or in deploring other people's sins. If external circum-stances cut off a woman's opportunities of feeling the emotion of tenderness and carry-ing out its behaviour for children of her own, her maternal instinct may drive her to lavish tenderness on other things—perhaps on a cat or a parrot, perhaps more usefully on some of the multitude of children and other people who are in need of loving help.

This finding of a new outlet for the be-haviour of an instinct may be called a

" deflection " of the instinct. Thus we may say that the unmarried woman showing unusual love for a domestic animal or for unfortunate persons is deflecting her maternal instinct to them. In using this word " deflection " we are suggesting the picture of a stream which can be deflected into one channel or another at will. That is as good a picture as any of the others we have used.

All such pictures are in danger of misleading us if we take them too seriously, but they are helpful to clearness of thought in psychology. It is best to use several different illustrations so that we may avoid being misled by any of them. Some things that are true of an instinct may, for example, not be true of a weed with a tap-root, but may be true of a leaking boiler or of a dammed-up stream. We must use our illustrations with discretion.

A deflection of an instinct may, of course, be a good thing, a bad thing, or neither bad nor good. If your cutting off of the ordinary outlets of anger leads you to write abusive anonymous letters, that will be thoroughly undesirable and it would have been better if you had let out your instinct of pugnacity in the ordinary way. If it leads you to carry on a war of extermination against the slugs in your garden, that will be a deflection which is good or bad according to whether you look at it from the point of view of the garden or of the slugs. If it leads you to engage more actively in the war against disease, so that your anger is called out by the existence of preventable disease, and you do valuable research work on the origin of cancer, or give money for furthering cancer research, your deflection will undoubtedly be a very good thing. Your instinct of pugnacity will have been deflected into channels of high social usefulness.

It is usual to give a separate name to the kind of deflection of instinct which is socially desirable and to call it a " sublimation." Thus one would be said to be sublimating one's instinct of pugnacity in cancer-research, but not in writing anonymous letters. A single woman who adopted an orphan child would be said to be " sublimating " her maternal instinct, but not one who gave her tenderness to a tame parrot. If we want a parallel to sublimation in our pictorial analogies, we shall have to imagine that the leak having been stopped up in our boiler, the steam is led to the piston so that its pressure disappears in doing useful work, or that the water of the dammed-up stream has been led to a water-wheel.

It was so common at one time for writers on psychology to neglect the existence of the instincts and to treat such emotional conditions as anger, fear, etc., as nothing but acquired habits, that the pendulum has now swung rather far the other way. Many writers suggest that all cutting off of the outlet of an instinct in one direction must necessarily mean that the same instinct will find an exactly equivalent outlet in some other direction. If this were altogether true, it would follow that reducing the number of times you lost your temper with other people must always be followed by a proportional increase of the anonymous letters you wrote or of the slugs you killed, or of energy you devoted to the discovery of the origin of cancer. Similarly it would follow that increasing the number of times you lost your temper would be followed by a proportional decrease in all these other activities.

It should be clear that this is an exaggeration of a true principle. While it is true that if you cut off the head of a perennial weed, it will sprout again from the root, it is also true that if you go on cutting off the new heads, the root itself will be weakened and will finally die. It is the same with instincts. If you make a habit of giving way to violent anger, your whole capacity for violence and anger will increase. On the other hand, checking the expression of anger at various outlets will tend to weaken your capacity for pugnacity. It is not that the energy behind an instinct is indestructible, but only that it is much more easily deflected than destroyed. If we are dissatisfied with our present emotional dispositions (if, for example, we are always giving way to anger directed towards the persons around us) it is generally easier and more efficient to attempt a wise deflection than to aim at the total destruction of the instinct concerned.

No true psychological teaching about the nature of instinct lends support to the singularly fatuous doctrine that : " Human nature never changes." Even the instincts themselves (the general tendencies to anger, fear, love, etc.), although inborn and rooted in the constitution of our nervous and endocrine gland systems, are not quite unchangeable.

But much more amenable to our will to change them, are the particular things which we hate, or fear, or love. These are determined by emotional habits which are, as it were, built on the foundations of our instincts. These emotional habits (or " sentiments ") are of far more practical importance to us in our adult life than are the instincts on which they are founded. You will find generally that it is the possibility of controlling such emotional habits which people are concerned to deny when they repeat the formula that " human nature never changes."

In truth, we not only can but must control our emotional habits. We cannot choose to be born without the capacity for anger. The constitution of our nervous systems and of our endocrine glands has settled that for us. But we can choose whether we shall be angry at, let us say, the inhabitants of certain other European countries or at the fact that a considerable number of the children in our own country are not able to get enough to eat. In the same way, we can choose whether to be afraid of bogey-men or of tuberculosis germs.

The fact that it is easier to deflect an instinct into a new channel than it is to cut it off altogether is not, however, the only reason why the wisest way to deal with an undesirable mode of expression of an instinct is to look for a desirable deflection. It has been shown that the origin of many of the illnesses which are popularly called " nervous " diseases is the condition of stress set up by allowing an instinct no outlet at all. Hysteria is an example of such a " nervous " complaint.

We know now that the word " nervous " in this connection is inaccurate. These complaints have nothing to do with the physical nerves—that is, with the slender grey fibres which carry impulses to and from the brain. They are failures of the mind or rather of the personality as a whole to adjust itself satisfactorily to a condition of mental stress. The scientific name for such a disorder is " psychoneurosis," and the persons suffering from these disorders are called " psychoneurotics." The condition of a psychoneurotic person resembles that of a steam engine when you have stopped up the leak without giving the steam access to the piston or any other method of escape. The pressure of the steam will go on increasing until the boiler blows up.

The ideal cure of the psychoneurotic is to give her (or him) some useful outlet for the bottled-up instincts. If a woman develops hysteria through the damming up of her sex-instinct, her symptoms will probably be relieved if the tenderness denied outlet in the normal channels of love for husband and children can be given to some other object. If, for example, she can give the self-sacrificing devotion of love to an adopted child or to some charitable cause, she will probably get better.

This cure will, in fact, generally not be so easy as it sounds. The hysteric is not merely a person who through external causes is not able to give love. There are also generally peculiarities in her character which prevent her from giving love, and no cure is possible until these peculiarities are to some extent overcome. Some of these peculiarities are probably inherited, while others have been acquired during her life-time and must be overcome by the special technical methods of psycho-analysis which can only be employed by a person (usually a doctor) with special training and qualifications.

It is not, however, with these disorders that we are now specially concerned. What

90

is of more practical importance to most of us is to bear in mind the fact that a satisfactory and socially allowable outlet for our instinctive tendencies is the best preventative of psychoneurosis for the mentally unstable and for the conditions of unhappiness and mental unrest which may be the result of the damming up (or repression) of instincts in the person of sound mind. Both idleness and unsatisfactory conditions of work are likely to be unfavourable to mental health, because in both the energies of the instincts may not be actively engaged in the business of living.

The remedy is not, of course, to give free rein to all the impulses of our instincts whether socially permitted or not. Although this is a popular misrepresentation of a certain side of modern psychological teaching, no psychologist or psychotherapist has ever taught anything so ridiculous. Apart from any moral objections, such an ideal would be quite impossible of realisation, for our different instincts would come into severe conflict with each other. You could not give way to all the violence dictated by your anger without a drastic repression of the impulses of your sympathy (which is just as instinctive as anger). There would therefore be psychological obstacles to your giving way freely to all the impulses of your instinct of pugnacity quite apart from the external difficulty that such conduct would quickly land you in prison.

The requirements of other people (who have as good a right to live their own lives as we have to live ours) and the requirements of the country's laws set limits to the ways in which our instincts can be allowed to express themselves. Each man's problem is so to dispose of his instincts within those limits that he achieves the maximum mental harmony (and consequently of mental efficiency and of happiness). Whenever, for some reason, he is unable to allow any instinct its normal satisfaction, or when for some reason this satisfaction must be delayed, he will try to find some way of deflecting it. Suitable deflections may be found in such activities as athletic sports, artistic or literary production, or perhaps some other form of work.

It must be remembered too that the condition under which painful (or even dangerous) mental stress is set up is not simply the damming up an instinctive line of behaviour; it is above all the damming up of an instinct after the instinct has gained strength by indulgence. The pressure in a pipe carrying water may not be very great if the pipe is kept permanently closed at one end; if, however, you allow the water to flow through the pipe and then suddenly close it, you set up a state of pressure which may burst the pipe. In the same way, you are not likely to suffer from much mental stress through never giving way to anger, but if you freely indulge your anger and then try to stop it, mental stress may be set up which makes the finding of a suitable deflection for your instinct of pugnacity an urgent necessity. This is much more obviously true of the sex instinct.

Peculiarly fortunate, of course, is the man who can find a satisfactory channel of sublimation in the work by which he earns his living. It is a special difficulty of our industrial civilisation that so many people are engaged in work so dull and unconstructive as to make this impossible. You will remember the war-time story of a private soldier who was reported by his sergeant-major to the company officer because he was not putting his heart into his work. The officer's inquiry as to what the work was received the reply that the man had to pick up pieces of paper with a pin stuck into the end of a stick. The man would have been poor indeed in his equipment of primitive instincts if he could have found a satisfactory channel of sublimation in such an activity. This is true also of too many of the tasks of peace time.

People sometimes ask what precisely must be done in order to sublimate an instinct. This is a reasonable and a very necessary question. Many of the extremely vague directions to " sublimate your instincts " with which one meets, are rather like telling a man to go to Jericho, without telling him what road he must start along and where he must turn to the right and where to the left. Detailed information of precisely what mental or bodily activities one is to carry out, is very generally omitted in references to " sublimation," and without such details general exhortations to sublimate are of little use.

This detailed advice must, of course, often be different for different individual cases. We can, however, give a few examples of the kind of thing it would be. Sometimes it is sufficient, when the natural outlet of an instinct is stopped, for the person concerned

94

simply to apply himself vigorously to some other activity. Thus a young man disappointed in love may find that when he applies himself to football or to the running of a boys' club, the pain of his disappointment lessens and that as it lessens there is an increasing amount of mental energy behind his play or his organisation of the club. Without much difficulty, he has effected a satisfactory sublimation.

Sometimes, however, more specific methods are required. I remember a tutor's advice to a student whose life and work were suffering from the disturbing effects of a love which could not by any possibility be satisfied. His advice was : " Whenever you feel yourself becoming sentimental about X. start applying yourself hard to your work." In the same way another person, whenever he felt his temper rising, instead of giving way to violent action or language against the person causing him annoyance, might go into the garden and kill slugs until the slaughter of slugs made his anger die down.

The final result of persistence in such behaviour would be that the emotional state of dissatisfaction (of love in the first case, and of anger in the second) would appear in consciousness as an impulse to work and to kill slugs respectively. In the end the emotional strain would be completely removed by successful application to these activities. Then the sublimation would be complete.

Sometimes this end might be attained by thought instead of by action, but this, I think, would prove a less easy method. If, whenever you felt anger, you made yourself think ferociously of slugs, you would no doubt find in the end that your pugnacity was deflected into the slug-killing channel. Action, however, is to be preferred to thought when action is possible. Effective action, however, in the new direction is not always possible when the impulse wells up. If, for example, we found our anger rising at our neighbour in the middle of a dinner party, it would not be practicable to leave the table and go out to kill slugs in our host's garden. Thought in the new direction, on the other hand, is nearly always possible.

Perhaps the most important of all reasons why instincts should be deflected into socially desirable channels is that so much socially desirable work remains to be done, while so much mental energy which might be put into the doing of it is wasted in other directions. It is difficult to imagine what good results might follow if a quarter of the anger wasted in war or in internal strife were directed against such evils as poverty, bad housing, disease, and smoke; or if a quarter of the tenderness wasted in misdirected sex-activity were directed towards the sick and the destitute. All this wasted energy might long ago have set human society on the road to a condition of social efficiency from which the avoidable miseries and injustices of the present order would appear like a bad dream.

LET us imagine a large public hall filled with people of all kinds. On a raised platform at the end of the hall stands one man—a lecturer or a political speaker. He is the one person in the hall who is in a prominent position. All the others are, from the point of view of the meeting, so unimportant as to be negligible, although they may, in other places and at other times, be much more important persons than the speaker. For the moment, however, the speaker alone dominates the hall. If any of the persons present were asked what was happening in the meeting at any moment, they would reply by describing what the speaker was saying or doing at the time, and not what the lady in the front row was saying to her neighbour or what the programme-seller was doing. In the meeting, the speaker alone matters and everyone else has sunk into a relatively insignificant position.

This is a picture of a mind in a condition

of " concentration." One outside object, one line of thought, or one task that is being performed, is alone occupying an important position in the mind. The multitude of other impressions from the outside world or of thoughts from the mind itself are kept in relative insignificance. They are not allowed to interfere with the one main thing with which the mind is occupied.

There may, for example, be many persons talking in a room. We can hear them all, but we can single out one conversation amongst the many and make it alone prominent in our minds. We say that we are " listening " to this one conversation which we have selected to concentrate on. It is not necessarily the loudest or even the most interesting. We have the power to take any of the sounds assailing our ears and give it this central position. In the same way, of all the objects of sight, we can choose to " watch " only one.

A public meeting of the kind we have described would clearly be the most efficient kind of gathering for most of the purposes for which people do meet together in public halls. Suppose now that we imagine a meeting of a very different kind at which every member of the audience interrupted at will. Such a meeting will be very inefficient. The speaker will get on only slowly, and may not be able to deliver his lecture or speech at all.

This is a picture of the common condition of mind-wandering or distractibility. Some people are unable to concentrate because, as soon as they attempt to put one thought into the dominant position, other thoughts force their way into prominence, by their interest or by their mere insistence. Such a person is trying, let us say, to read a difficult book, but is unable to grasp its meaning because his mind is simultaneously repeating the words of a song he heard yesterday, considering whether to buy a new pair of boots, hoping that it will be fine to-morrow, picturing where he will go for a walk if it is, and wondering whether he forgot to wind up the clock in the front room last night.

This is a condition into which we all pass when we are suffering from mental fatigue through having already carried out as much concentrated mental effort as is good for us. Nature has many devices for preventing us from exhausting our brains. Some people always (and all of us sometimes) find, how-

103

ever, that the mere effort to begin to concentrate makes them pass into this condition
of mind-wandering, even when there can be
no question of mental fatigue. For people
afflicted in this way, there is clear necessity
for some kind of mental discipline which will
increase their power of concentration.

Most systems of mental development do,
in fact, attach a good deal of importance to
concentration. Books on mental development sometimes have as their titles the one
word " concentration." The various Yoga
systems of the East used methods of meditation far more arduous than any we are ever
likely to be tempted to carry out ourselves,
at the end of which those who used them were
able to hold one thought steadily in the mind
without distraction.

We may remind ourselves of a general
principle which we laid down in the first
chapter of this book. It would be absurd
to pursue concentration as an end in itself.
If it is to be practised at all it must be because
it can be justified by its contribution to
mental efficiency. In what way is concentration necessary to mental efficiency ?

The real practical reason why we want this
power of concentration is because it is essential

in all kinds of learning, mental and muscular. If we want to learn a poem, or to learn what Einstein thinks about space and time, or to learn a new movement in a game, there is only one efficient way of doing it. That way is to have what is to be learnt in the focus of attention and all irrelevant and distracting things excluded from the mind.

There are some movements which we cannot learn to control simply because we cannot by any amount of effort bring them into the field of attention. The beating of the heart is an example. Breathing, on the other hand, can either be controlled or go on automatically, because we can at will bring the movements of breathing into the field of attention although they are ordinarily outside it. The movements of the muscles of the heart cannot be brought into consciousness in the same way. It seems to be theoretically possible that by a special training of the power of attention it could. The Hatha-Yogis of India claim that by their method of training the power of concentration, they can bring the beating of the heart under willed control. It seems very probable, and the only reason for regarding this fact as of no more than theoretical interest is that there seems to be no practical advantage to be gained from controlling the beating of one's heart.

Similarly, an American professor has recently been showing how it is possible to teach people voluntarily to move their ears by bringing this group of muscles into the field of attention. Again this is of no practical value (although it is said to be an effective drawing-room trick). Its interest lies in the illustration of the principle that new muscular movements can be learned as soon as the movements of the muscles can be made the subject of concentrated attention. An important practical application of this principle is in the teaching of singing and of phonetics, when the pupil is taught to give his attention to and so to control previously unconscious movements of the tongue and larynx.

While the various tasks of learning require concentration, they are not the only purposes for which we require this attitude of mind. Any task which is being performed for the first time or that involves new problems can only be carried out efficiently if attention is concentrated on it. Without concentration, one could not play chess, or conduct a business, or sustain an argument, or do any bit of hard efficient thinking. Inability to concentrate is, therefore, a serious loss, and the highly distractible persons whose minds wander whenever they try to get down to a task are suffering from serious mental inefficiency. We cannot be surprised at the prominent position which concentration takes in all systems which claim to teach methods of increasing mental powers.

We can hardly fail to notice that there are two very different processes by which the mind can pass to a condition of concentration on one thing. If you see a street accident, it will at once occupy the focus of attention and all other impressions of all kinds will fade into insignificance. Your attention will be concentrated on the accident. This concentration takes place in a very different way from the effort you make in learning something by heart. The first is spontaneous. The accident has concentrated your attention on it by its own interest; no effort of yours has been necessary. The concentration in learning by heart, on the other hand, is deliberate; it is the result of willed effort. Like all effort, the effort required to maintain deliberate concentration is fatiguing. If it goes on for a long time we feel tired and our minds begin to wander.

It is an obvious advantage in learning that the concentration on the thing to be learned should be, as far as possible, spontaneous and effortless, because then the task of learning will be least fatiguing. It is the business of every teacher and of every writer to present his subject-matter in as interesting a way as possible, so that very little effort is necessary on the part of his hearers or readers for them to keep their mind concentrated on it.

Yet, as a matter of fact, very few indeed of the things that are worth learning are so interesting that attention is concentrated on to them quite spontaneously. A good many things that we want to learn and a good many of the tasks we want to perform are so uninteresting that a great deal of effort is required in order to keep the mind concentrated on them. No one would ever learn a new language or write a book, if he trusted entirely to the power of the interest of his task to attach his attention to it continually. He must, on the contrary, make himself carry out the task he has started by a sustained effort of deliberate attention.

Since some of our tasks must necessarily require effort in concentration, the power of willed concentration is one which must be developed if we are deficient in it. There is only one way in which this capacity can be developed, and that is the obvious one—by practice. This means that there is one very important exception to the rule that any learning task should be made as interesting as possible; this exception is when it is being learned not for its own sake, but as an exercise in concentration. This does not mean that in order to practise concentration, one should learn something useless or unpleasant. It is better to acquire the ability to concentrate by learning a poem by heart and so acquiring something of permanent value, or by carrying out an operation delightful in itself (such as chess or draughts).

The Buddhists increase their powers of concentration by a discipline of continually holding the image of some indifferent object (such as a lump of clay) steadily in the mind until it can think of that alone. In the same way, children used to be taught by heart the names of the capes round the coast of England (perhaps they are still). This was clearly an exercise in concentration, since the matter learned was of no value in itself. If the children, when grown up, ever wanted to navigate the coast of England, it would be necessary for them to buy a reliable chart and not trust to their memories. I have already mentioned one writer on mind-training who invites his readers to hold the image of a chair steadily in their minds for a long time.

We shall be right to follow the Buddhists and the educators, and the gentleman of the chair, in using deliberate practice as a method of improving the power to concentrate and of eliminating mind-wandering. We shall be wise, however, to modify their methods by remembering that concentration may as well be practised on something useful as on something useless. It will be better to learn poems by heart, to study mathematics, or to master a new language, than to burden our memories with the capes round the coast of England, or with the images of chairs. A practical exercise for those who find themselves deficient in the ability to concentrate would be to learn a certain number of lines of poetry every day.

There are a few points about the connection of bodily posture with concentration which are worth noticing. A position in which the muscles are braced up is one favourable to concentration. If we are to do a job demanding real concentrated attention, we shall be better able to accomplish it sitting in a hard-backed chair than lounging in an arm-chair.

At the same time, it must be remembered that keeping the muscles tense is not the same thing as mental concentration and is not even essential to it, and it has the objection that it is fatiguing in itself. Many people think they are concentrating when they are really doing nothing except keeping many of their bodily muscles, such as those of the forehead and face, in a state of uselessly fatiguing contraction. This muscular contraction (which is very obvious amongst children and people unaccustomed to mental work) ought to be eliminated because it is unnecessarily tiring. Mental concentration can be carried on perfectly efficiently with muscles relaxed. Some great thinkers, as, for example, Descartes, have managed to work very efficiently in bed.

Different people differ very much in their power of quickly taking up an attitude of concentrated attention and of returning to it

111

when it has been disturbed by the necessity of breaking off one task for a short time in order to attend to another. Working with frequent interruptions can never be a very efficient way of carrying out concentrated work, but since all of us must sometimes attend to other things during periods when we wish to work, the power of rapidly reassuming the attitude of concentration after interruption is also worth cultivating.

Much more important is the power of concentrating in the presence of outside distractions. It is quite possible to concentrate efficiently while a great deal of noise is going on, even the noise of other persons talking, so long as no one talks to you. Experiment shows, in fact, that concentrated learning may be more efficient in the presence of outside noise, presumably because the presence of a possible source of distraction forces us to make a greater effort of concentration. The mental worker who insists that he can only read or write in a house which is absolutely quiet is a great nuisance to other people, and should realise that he is merely giving evidence of an inefficient and imperfectly trained mind. If he cannot concentrate in the presence of noises which do not concern him, he should learn to do so as soon as he can.

We must never forget that concentration is not the only useful attitude of attention. It is useful for some things, but bad for others. Sometimes an attitude of mind is required in which more things than one are maintained in an important position of the mind. This is necessary, for example, when you are driving a motor-car or crossing the street. For these tasks, a concentrated attention would be just as dangerous as a condition of pure mind-wandering. The attitude required is that of " distributed attention."

Distributed attention may be compared to a kind of public gathering in which the platform is occupied by many persons acting together—let us say an orchestra, or a group of actors performing a play. There is still a platform and the arrangement of persons on it is not haphazard, but the platform is no longer occupied by one person. Indeed any one person on the platform who pushes himself into a too prominent position will spoil the effectiveness of the whole group.

We all know the kind of driver of a motor-car who applies concentrated attention to his task. He keeps his eyes fixed rigidly on the part of the road immediately in front of him and grips his steering handle hard. If a chicken appears on the road a hundred yards ahead, that chicken becomes firmly fixed in the focus of his attention, while he ignores pedestrians on his left, the cyclists in front of him, and the motor lorry bearing down on him from a side road. Nothing but luck saves him from a serious accident every time he takes his car out. He generally considers himself a careful driver, but he is in reality a very bad one. He is bringing concentrated attention to bear on a task which can only be efficiently performed by distributed attention.

A similar distribution of attention is necessary when one is crossing a crowded road. The motor-car approaching on one side must not so occupy the mind that all the other possible dangers of the road are ignored. All must have their place on the platform of attention.

A person who uses concentrated attention for driving a car or for crossing a road is using his mind as inefficiently as the man who tries to solve a problem or learn a poem with distributed attention, and, on the whole, the results of the former mistake are likely to be the more serious. It is worse to be run over than to fail to learn a poem.

In order to have our powers of attention efficiently under control, it is not, however, enough simply to cultivate the power of being able to concentrate and to distribute our attention. There is also a condition of attention which is the exact opposite of concentration—that of mental relaxation. This is when no effort is made to keep any impressions in the position of honour, but in which all have an equal liberty to force themselves to the forefront of our minds.

Is this to be regarded simply as a condition of mental inefficiency, or has it a value of its own? Undoubtedly, it too has its value in the right place. It is of no use for any kind of work, but it has value for rest. This condition of relaxed attention reaches its culminating point in sleep, when impressions from outside things are ignored altogether or merely woven into the fabric of our dreams.

We have compared the concentrated mind to a meeting addressed by one man, and the mind in distributed attention to the performance of a play. A mind in relaxed attention would be like a purely social gathering. In such a gathering everyone has equal rights,

115

but the whole character of the gathering is destroyed as soon as one person pushes himself to the front or talks in such a loud voice that he attracts the notice of everyone. Such gatherings can hardly have the ordinary criteria of efficiency applied to them. They are pleasant enough recreations, but they are not meant to be meetings to perform any work.

The power of relaxation also deserves to be cultivated. We cannot work all the time. The efficient worker is the man who, when his task is over, can leave his mind free to occupy itself as it will. The man who still thinks of his work when his work is over is like a spring which is always under tension. He is not a really efficient mental worker.

Probably the main reason for the use of alcohol by moderate drinkers is that it enables them to accomplish this end of relaxation. The experiments which prove that one works less efficiently mentally and physically after taking alcohol, always seem to me to be irrelevant to the real point. Certainly alcohol reduces efficiency in work, and this is always recognised by mental workers although not always by physical workers. It interferes with work just because it accomplishes this end of relaxation. Its justification (if it has any) must be sought in its value for the promotion of the relaxed attitude of mind. Its service is to rest, not to work.

I am not, of course, defending the use of alcohol but merely pointing out why it is used. It must be admitted that although alcohol helps relaxation, it has many bad effects. In any case, we do not want to be dependent on a drug for effective relaxation. If we have so cultivated our mental powers that we can relax at will, we are better off than the man who is dependent on his wine. Besides, the willed control of relaxation is cheaper.

If we want to develop the power of relaxing mental tension at will, this too can be made into a mental exercise which can be carried out at intervals between mental work. It will be an advantage, as we have already seen, to relax the muscles of our bodies, since this in itself has a tendency to induce the condition of mental relaxation. This may be done in a comfortable chair. While relaxing the muscles deliberately relax the tension of the mind. With as little effort as possible refuse to allow it to be engrossed by fatiguing problems which are the subjects of its activity while it is at work. Allow it to occupy itself restfully with the day-dreams that will come to you. These dreams, like alcohol, have no value for work, but they have value for rest. By practising deliberate relaxation in this way, the power of relaxing at will can be brought under willed control. The man who has achieved this control can rest efficiently as well as work efficiently.

For efficiency in mental work, the ability to concentrate is undoubtedly of the very first importance, and it is an ability which can be improved by deliberate practice. Nobody doubts the value of concentration, even though not everyone is willing to make the effort necessary to escape from inefficient habits of mind-wandering in mental work. The danger is rather that we should make a fetish of concentration. The really efficient mind is the mind that can not only concentrate, but can also distribute attention for tasks demanding distributed attention and can relax efficiently when its tasks are over.

IT sometimes happens that when one is travelling in a railway train, one finds oneself sitting opposite to a dignified gentleman who obviously holds some administrative position in the public services. He puts down his paper, and begins to address one in such terms as these : " Perfectly scandalous, these miners. Wanting a seven-hour day indeed ! I wish I could have a seven-hour day. I frequently have to work for fourteen hours or more in the day."

The psychologist might reply as follows : " Let us suppose that what you are saying is strictly accurate, and that you do frequently work for fourteen hours a day or more. There are two alternatives. Either these long hours of work are your fault, or they are not. If they are not, I am sorry for you. If, on the other hand, they are your fault, you ought to be ashamed of admitting that you are guilty of such a very inefficient method of working.

" For at least the last six of those fourteen hours you must be working in a condition of extreme fatigue, a condition in which not only is the work very unpleasant for you, but it is very badly performed. No doubt your temper during those last six hours is abominable, and both your subordinates and your wife are made to suffer by it. You work slowly and find that much of the work that is done one day will have to be done again the next. When you go to bed you are so tired you cannot sleep properly. You therefore go to your office the next morning even more fatigued than the day before, and this condition gets worse until finally your health breaks down.

" Although you may not be willing to admit it even to yourself, you probably take a certain pride in having broken down through over-work. When you tell people the cause of your illness there is a ring in your voice which suggests that you are thanking God that you are not as other men, even as these miners. You go away for a long and expensive holiday and come back at the end of a few months and start the process over again.

" It is possible that it is not your fault,

so I give you my sympathy, but in any case your satisfaction in the process is entirely misplaced. Avoidable indulgence in the poisonous products of over-fatigue is no more creditable than over-indulgence in strong drink. You would not be proud to say that you had performed your work in your office inefficiently and had finally had to take a long holiday because you had been drinking too much. You should feel no more satisfaction in the same result having followed from the fact that you have worked too much."

In this matter of work and rest we might all of us take a lesson from some of the most indefatigable and efficient workers that we can ever meet with, the muscles of our heart. Unless we are foolish and impose a severe, continuous strain on these muscles we find that they do not over-work themselves. They contract, driving the blood through the arteries and veins, and after each contraction there is a small fraction of time during which they rest. This rest period is just long enough for them to get rid of the fatigue which has resulted from their previous contraction and so enables them to contract efficiently again. If your heart muscles decided to take a long rest because they had over-worked themselves, you would die. You would not think that your heart had done something to be proud of. There is no likelihood of this happening, however. The heart muscles of ordinary healthy people are not so foolish.

Let us be clear about the fact that over-work, whether thrust on us from outside or carried out by our own choice, is inefficient. Manual workers were severely over-worked in the early part of the nineteenth century in England, when even little children were working for fourteen and more hours a day. This system was not only brutal; it was also uneconomic. When a bill was introduced into parliament to shorten the workers' day from fourteen hours to twelve hours, the manufacturers cried out that all their profits would be lost because they needed twelve hours' work from their employees in order to pay the costs of production and on the last two hours alone they made profits.

It was found, however, that you do not reduce output by decreasing hours of work from fourteen to twelve. Such a decrease of hours may be followed (not immediately but in a short time) by an actual increase in the amount of work done every day. In the same way, it has been found that the actual output of work may be increased by reducing hours of work from twelve to ten and even from ten to eight. Of course, this process cannot go on indefinitely. If the number of hours worked in a day is sufficiently reduced a time comes when further reduction of hours will cause a reduction in output of work.

To many people it seems as obvious as it did to the nineteenth-century manufacturers that more work will be done in a working day of fourteen hours than in one of twelve, while the opposite assertion seems to them to be absurd. Yet a little reflection will show that this proposition is less obvious than appears at first sight. No motorist supposes that he will get a greater mileage out of a gallon of petrol by spreading its consumption over three hours instead of two. In fact he will probably get less.

We are inclined to think of a man's output of work as a stream which flows at a constant rate, so we can get twice as much of it by tapping it for double the time. But suppose it were really a constant total amount each day, this would no longer be true. Taking it out for double the time would mean that we got the same quantity at half the speed, and there might be secondary bad effects of this which would actually reduce the total amount. A dairyman is not fool enough to suppose that he could get an indefinitely large quantity of milk by milking his cows all day long, instead of only at the usual times.

The fact that a reduction of excessive hours of work may be followed by an increase of work performed is one that has been established again and again by careful observation. The reason is really a perfectly simple one. Let us suppose that a man is working for eight hours every day. While he is at work, fatigue is gradually set up by the accumulation in his blood of the chemical substances produced by his muscles while they are at work. During his night's rest these substances disappear and he gets up in the morning fresh and unfatigued.

Now let us suppose that his hours of work are suddenly changed to ten hours a day. He will start his first ten-hour day perfectly fresh and may therefore do as much work during the first eight hours of those ten as he previously did in the previous eight-hour day, and what he does in the next two hours (which will be nearly but not quite a quarter of his previous work) will produce an increase of output. It might, therefore, be imagined that increasing his hours of work has increased his output.

So it has for the time, but at the end of ten hours' work he is much more fatigued than he used to be at the end of his eight-hour day. Since we supposed that his night's rest was just enough to overcome his fatigue from an eight-hour day, it will be insufficient to overcome his fatigue from a ten-hour day. He will start his next day's work still in a slightly fatigued condition, and his rate of work will, therefore, be slower through the whole day. His second ten-hour day will, therefore, produce a smaller increase of output than his first (and perhaps none at all). It will also leave him even more tired at the end than he was the day before. His night's rest will be still more inadequate to remove this tiredness, and he will start his third day more tired than he started his second, so that his rate of work will be still slower.

This process will go on until his rate of work is so slow during the whole day that his actual output through the ten-hour day will be less than that of the eight-hour day. At the same time he will always be more tired and, therefore, less happy at his work, more liable to accidents, and producing more spoiled work.

If, in the same way, you now shorten his day's work to eight hours, his recovery will not be a sudden one. His first eight-hour day will start with the fatigue left by his previous ten-hour days, so his output for that day must necessarily be less than it was during the previous day when he worked for ten hours. There will be, to begin with, a fall in output as a result of decreasing his hours of work, but this again is only for a time. As he recovers from the condition of chronic fatigue which has resulted from his over-work, his rate of work will increase until during the eight-hour day he is actually able to produce more than he previously could in his ten-hour day.

I am, of course, only taking eight and ten hours as examples. The actual number of hours' work which will just be compensated for by a night's rest will depend on the nature of the work. Also, I am not suggesting that workers should be required to work until they can just recover from the effects of their work by a night's rest. The worker may reasonably say that he does not want to devote the last ounce of his energy to his daily labour; and that in a prosperous country one of the social goods that we should aim at is a working day which is short enough to make it possible for the workers to devote time and energy to interests outside their work.

What has been discovered about efficient hours of labour in the workshop may very well be applied in the direction of our own studies or other activities in which we can choose our own times of work. The length of the most efficient working day is, of course, different for different tasks. A man might paint spots on a rocking-horse for a much longer day than he could carry bars of pig-iron. An eight-hour day has been found to be too long for maximum output in some parts of the very delicate work of scientific instrument makers.

Five hours is probably as long as can be spent profitably in one day in pure study. Students spend much longer than this in study just before their examinations, but it is most likely that what is read after five hours of work is not effectively retained.

One whose work is only partly study, while he is also engaged in administrative duties and a certain amount of office routine, may work for many hours longer without any loss of efficiency.

School children are given home-work which, with their hours in school, gives them a total length of hours of study longer even than an adult would find it possible to engage in intellectual work. If we suggest that school hours should be reduced, we are suspected of wishing to encourage idleness. The child, of course, does not break down. His protective mechanism against over-fatigue prevents him from paying concentrated attention during these long hours. The care of foolish adults to protect him from the dangers of idleness, produces, therefore, the very habit of inattentiveness and mind-wandering during intellectual work which will be a curse to him in all his later intellectual efforts. It is also liable to have the unfortunate effect of producing a distaste for study.

It will be only the very foolish who will misunderstand what has been said here, so much as to suppose that it is in praise of idleness. Idleness, or the failure to put into

130

our work all the physical and mental energy we can, is so obviously a source of inefficiency that it is hardly necessary to call attention to its evils. Those who are habitually idle are idle through moral weakness and not because they suppose it an efficient thing to be.

Nor am I suggesting that we ought to stop work when we feel tired. The feeling of tiredness can easily arise when there is no real fatigue, and may only mean that we are not interested in our work. One of the temptations of mental work is to stop not when we are fatigued but when we begin to be bored. Boredom may feel very much like fatigue; it may produce headache, mind-wandering, etc. The difference is that boredom can and must be overcome by strenuous willed effort.

Over-work does not mean working when you are fatigued. That is often done in sports without any harm resulting to the person whose heart is sound. The mountain climber is often in a condition of physical exhaustion, which would be a great evil if it were the permanent condition in which he did his daily work. On the mountains it is no evil, but is a valuable training for character. The ability to endure fatigue, hunger and cold in the pursuit of sport is a safeguard against the development of that softness of character of which idleness is one symptom.

Over-work does not mean working when you are fatigued; it means habitually working more than your night's rest enables you to recover from. That is a much more complicated thing. Public men (bishops and statesmen) are fond of telling us that hard work is a good thing. That is undoubtedly true. They go on to say that no man has ever been harmed by over-work. That is a deadly lie. The very same public men who preach the glories of over-work preach a more edifying sermon when they themselves break down in health and take several months' holiday as a result of their inefficient habit of working too long.

It is impossible to guess how many wars and strikes have been precipitated through statesmen coming to responsible decisions when they are in the condition of irritability brought about by over-fatigue. In a national crisis the patriotic statesman gladly sacrifices his own night's sleep so that he may spend the whole night in conferences and negotiations. Then on the following day there is a sudden rupture which to the outside observer bears all the marks of unreasoning bad temper on both sides due to nervous exhaustion. The patriotic statesman would be ashamed to sleep when the affairs of the nation required his unceasing vigilance, but it would often be better for the nation if he did.

It is true, of course, that circumstances may arise in which over-work is necessary. The public men who have broken down in health through over-work, have often done it through no fault of their own. Their only fault is the speeches they have made in praise of excessive work. Whether it be necessary or not, however, nature sternly exacts her penalty for over-work. For a sufficiently good cause we must be prepared to pay that penalty, but let us make no mistake about what the penalty is. Spending too long hours at work decreases, in the long run, the total amount of work we do. For every hour of over-work we must afterwards pay in compulsory rest far more hours than we have gained. The net result at the end will be a loss of work and not a gain. In order to work efficiently, we must also rest efficiently.

Resting does not, of course, necessarily mean remaining still. The brain worker who digs his garden in the evening may be resting more efficiently than he would by simply doing nothing at all. We are all resting by changing our kind of occupation when we take holidays, although our lives may then be full of strenuous and varied activities.

Of all methods of resting, however, the most important is sleep. No one can work efficiently who is suffering from sleeplessness. Sleeplessness may, of course, proceed from something which it is beyond the power of mental control to remove. If we suffer from sleeplessness as a result of indigestion, the remedy does not lie in the direction of mental exercises. The remedy is to stop eating indigestible things at supper. Similarly if we are kept awake by toothache, we must go to a dentist and have the tooth removed.

These are physical causes of sleeplessness, which must be treated by physical means. Sleeplessness may, however, have mental causes, such as worry, excitement, or even a simple conviction that one will not sleep.

Worry which is keeping one awake may, of course, have an outside cause. A man may be kept awake at night because he is worrying at the thought that he is not able to make enough money to pay the expenses of his house. The sleeplessness itself may be making it more difficult for him to meet his expenses because it decreases his earning power. The important thing for him to remember, however, is that it is not his approaching bankruptcy that keeps him awake, but his anxiety about it. His sleeplessness has really a mental and not a physical cause; it is of a kind that will yield to mental treatment.

It is with the removal of such mental causes of sleeplessness that we are specially concerned. We have already mentioned in an earlier chapter the use of auto-suggestion to produce sleep. This is one of the most important practical uses of the method of auto-suggestion. Continual repetition of the formula " I am falling asleep " will be found to induce sleep when all such methods as counting imaginary sheep jumping over hedges are found to be quite useless. If, however, we are strongly excited or anxious it is better to use auto-suggestion first to produce calm and afterwards use it to produce sleep.

It is a peculiarity of sleep that it takes

place easily only under accustomed circumstances. Most of us habitually go to bed and turn out the light and surround ourselves by quiet before sleeping and we are likely to find that we are unable to sleep if any of these conditions are not fulfilled. These conditions can be summed up as the absence of stimulation from outside. We sleep on comfortable beds so that we may not have sensations of pressure on the muscles and bones which we should feel if we slept on hard boards. We turn out the light so that our eyes may not be assailed by visual impressions, and we insist on quiet so that our ears may not be disturbed by auditory impressions.

In fact, however, this absence of stimulation from outside is not so necessary as is commonly supposed. It is quite possible to sleep comfortably on a hard board with lights burning and noises going on all round. Most of us did so many times during the war. It is a useful power to have even in peace time, for there are few of us who do not sometime want to sleep in a train, or in a room with other people, when we shall be neither in physical comfort nor in silence and darkness.

The development of this power is not difficult. What keeps us awake is not the outside light or noise, but our own action about it. It is for this reason that we are aroused at once by a question addressed to ourselves, while we can sleep calmly through the much louder noise of a train in which we are travelling. The reason we are kept awake by a conversation or other noise in the room in which we want to sleep is generally that we are trying to do something about it—we are trying to shut it out from our consciousness.

This suggests what is the true remedy for the disturbance of sleep from outside stimulations. Do not make the effort to shut them out from your mind, but passively allow them to make their entrance. If you try to exclude the noise of someone else talking while you are trying to sleep, you will find that you succeed only in keeping yourself awake. If, on the other hand, you listen calmly to the conversation, it will lull you to sleep. This is the surprising fact which has been discovered by everyone who has solved the problem of sleeping through outside disturbances.

I REMEMBER once reading a story about the examination of candidates for admission to a cadet college either of the army or navy. The boys were left in an ante-room before they went in for their final interview. At this interview, they were asked what objects were standing on the mantelpiece in the room they had just left. If they could answer correctly they were given high credit for their powers of observation.

This story illustrates a very common fallacy about memory. The person who devised this test obviously thought that there was some merit in remembering, quite apart from whether the things remembered were important or trivial. But this is absurd. None of us can possibly remember all the objects which meet us during the course of a day, and the mind that did so would have accomplished nothing useful, but merely cluttered itself up with useless memories. Our power of remembering is useful to us,

141

because it enables us to recall things whose recall will be serviceable to us. For this end, it is just as important that we should forget the trivial as that we should remember the important.

Most of us have in our houses a room which we use for papers, boxes, unseasonable clothes, and so on. What should we think of a man who put in his box-room everything that entered his house and destroyed nothing? We should not consider that he had a highly efficient box-room, because it would be so full of articles that were useless that its owner would be unable to find things when he really wanted them. It is the same with the mind. The well-ordered mind is the mind which remembers what it wants to remember and forgets what it has no need for remembering.

In all the useful remembering we do in our adult lives, this kind of selection is made. We just remember what we need and forget the rest. When I wrote the story with which this chapter begins, I had forgotten (and have still forgotten) the name of the newspaper from which I read it, the time at which I read it, the name of the college of which it was told, and the name of the writer who told it. All these were useless details. I had just remembered the one thing that I wanted, which was the story itself.

That, surely, is a more useful, as well as a more usual, way of remembering than that of the person who recalls the ornaments on a mantelpiece. When we read books (certainly if we read a large number) it is very necessary that we should forget a great part of them. No harm is done by this so long as we remember all that we shall afterwards need.

As a matter of fact, we are not at all likely to find ourselves burdened with this kind of gramophonic memory which forgets nothing. Our forgetting of the unimportant takes place automatically and efficiently and may, therefore, be left to take care of itself. Our difficulty is much more often that we forget too much, so that we want to train our power of remembering. How are we to do this?

The obvious answer to this question is to say that we can improve the memory by practice. By habitually performing tasks of remembering, we might reasonably hope to be able to improve our memories.

For once, however, this answer is shown by careful experiment not to be an adequate one. The trouble is that there is no one thing which we can call " the Memory." Remembering is a name we give to a whole group of different mental activities which happen to have the same practical result of recalling something which has gone before. Sometimes, when we are able to recall a fact about the past merely by reviving some habit formed in the parts of our bodies we use for speech (the larynx, tongue and lips), we say that we have remembered this fact. This, for example, is what is happening when we learn by heart the dates of the kings of England, and it is an important part of what is happening when we are learning a poem by heart.

Quite different from this is remembering by calling up a mental image. When we say that we remember the face of a friend, this simply means that we can call up before our mind's eye a mental image (that is, a mental picture) of his face.

Both of these kinds of remembering are quite different from what happens when we say that we can remember a lecture. In this case, it is unlikely that we can recall

144

either the actual words used by the lecturer or a mental picture of his appearance. We are merely able to recall the meaning of what he said. This is generally called " logical " memory to distinguish it from the other kinds of remembering which are called " mechanical " memory.

Now, which of all these different operations do we mean to improve when we try to practise our memories? If both were the operation of a single faculty of memory, it would be reasonable to expect that practice in learning by heart would improve our power of recalling the meaning of a lecture. But since in fact they are two quite distinct mental operations, we cannot be certain that practice in the one operation will at all help the other. It may, and, on the other hand, it may not.

We must notice too that the " mechanical " remembering of learning by heart is not, in itself, of much use to us in our adult life. It is very rarely indeed that it is necessary for us to learn anything by heart. What we do want is to be able to acquire the meaning of something—some lecture heard or book read—and for this purpose " mechanical " remembering is of no use.

K

In fact, it will be found, that practice in learning by heart only helps logical remembering in an indirect and limited way—by increasing our power of willed concentration. If what limits our power of remembering meanings is that we are not able to concentrate sufficiently, then we should practise learning by heart as described in Chapter V, until our power of willed concentration is improved.

The true way to increase our power of remembering is not to try to improve the " memory," but to begin to use more efficient methods of learning. One way of increasing the efficiency of our methods of learning is to learn with more concentrated attention.

The effect of auto-suggestion must also be remembered. It is not so much that one should use auto-suggestion as an aid to remembering itself (although this may sometimes be found useful), but it is necessary to bear in mind that unintended auto-suggestions may often cause forgetting. A confident attitude of mind is the best one to bring to a task of learning. If you say : " I have a bad memory, I shall never be able to remember this," you are unintentionally making an auto-suggestion that you will fail to remember, and this is quite likely to be effective in making you forget. The reason why many people forget what they try to learn is because they have already made up their minds that they will forget.

Systems for training the memory also generally include training for different kinds of imagery. Some things may be remembered by clear visual images (that is, mental pictures of things seen), others by clear auditory images (or representations to the mind's ear of things once heard). Visual images are not essential (although they are helpful) in enabling us to remember details of things that have been presented to the eyes. It is for this reason that a lecturer does not generally trust to his audience's power of remembering his words alone; he also tries to create visual images by drawing pictures on the black-board, or by illustrating his remarks with lantern slides.

In the same way, auditory images enable us to remember things heard. The person who has auditory imagery is enabled to recall before his mind pieces of music which he has once heard. The absence of auditory imagery must always prevent anyone from going very far in musical appreciation. Such a person may hear and enjoy pieces of music played in a concert, but when the concert is over they are gone from his mind and from his power of thinking about them until he actually hears them played again. He cannot reproduce them in his mind alone.

It is not certain how far one's power of imagery can be trained. Some experimenters have reported that, by deliberate practice in recalling things by visual imagery or by auditory imagery, they have increased their power of using these images. There is no reason for supposing that this process can go on indefinitely. Apparently some people are deficient and always will be deficient in visual imagery, while others are and always will be deficient in auditory imagery. Those of us, however, who are conscious of a failure in our memory which results from the absence of one kind of imagery, may help to make this failure less by practising that kind of imagery. Even more usefully, we can form the habit of using in our remembering those kinds of imagery which happen to be well developed in ourselves.

There are a few other points connected with the methods of learning which are worth noticing. Although it has been pointed out by psychologists for a very long time, it is not generally known what is the correct way of learning a long passage by heart. When we were children, we sometimes had to learn a chapter of the Bible by heart, or learn to say the speech of Mark Antony. We were usually taught to split it up into small bits and learn one bit every day and then string them all together at the end.

Experiments have proved that the best way to do a task like this (that is, the easiest and most effective way) is to repeat the whole passage every time and not to cut it up. Splitting a long passage into parts and learning them separately, involves unnecessary work, and what is learned is not so well retained as it would have been had the passage been learned from the beginning as a whole.

It is also not generally known that a task of learning is better performed if the repetitions are distributed in time. If you repeat a passage twelve times in succession, you will not have learnt it as well as if you had made the same number of repetitions with an interval of five minutes or an hour between them. It is as if what has been once repeated must be allowed to settle

149

down before it is repeated again. After the effects of the first repetition have settled down the next one is more effective.

For the same reason, a task of learning can be disturbed by another task being performed immediately after it. This is like driving traffic over a newly made road before it has become sufficiently strong to bear disturbance. After you have learned something difficult a lapse of say five minutes should be allowed before a new task is attempted. It has been proved by experiment that if you learn one thing and immediately afterwards learn something else, the result will be that the thing you have first learned will be largely forgotten.

It should also be remembered that learning is not carried on efficiently in a state of fatigue, simply because in this condition attention cannot be concentrated. It is a sheer waste of time to try to learn things at the end of a hard day if they can be as conveniently learned at the beginning. More time will be spent when you are tired and the learning will be less effective. This means that the time you can efficiently spend during a single day in pure learning is much shorter than the time you can spend in any other kind of activity. If hours in school were regulated by scientific principles, the time that children were supposed to spend in learning at school each day would be a great deal shorter than it is now.

Another feature which is common to most mind-training systems, is the practice of various more or less useful tricks for remembering. Some things are remembered more easily than others. A picture, for example, is impressed on the memory more easily than a number. When, therefore, it is necessary to learn numbers, it is useful to convert them into pictures. You may, for example, remember the number 26 by forming a picture of a plate of beef (beef beginning with the second letter of the alphabet and ending with the sixth), 27 may be remembered by the picture of a bog, 28 by a picture of a bath, and so on.

By using a code of pictures like this it is possible to perform feats of memory which would be quite impossible in any other way. There is, for example, a good parlour trick described and performed by Professor G. H. Thomson, in which you allow people to call out to you in rapid succession the name of a large number of different objects, such as rose, wind, bicycle, park, motor-car, and so on, up to the number of sixty or a hundred. Afterwards you undertake to tell them the position in the series of each particular object called out. You are able, let us say, to tell them that carpet was 67th on the list, and that candle was called out 25th.

The trick you use for this is that when " carpet " is called out to you, you form a mental picture of a frog sitting on a carpet (because frog is the mental picture for 67). In the same way when " candle " is called out you form a mental picture of a bee standing on the top of a candle. You make no particular effort to remember these pictures (it is not necessary), but you will find that when you are asked about the word carpet, the picture of a carpet with a frog sitting on it will come back to your mind, and you will then know that carpet was called out 67th. This is quite an easy trick for anyone to perform who has a reasonable command of visual imagery, and it is one which would be quite impossible by any other method. It illustrates the possibility of using devices of this kind to enable one to remember particular kinds of matter.

In the same way, it is found that sensible

material is learnt more easily than meaningless, and that poetry is learnt more easily
than prose. When, therefore, we want to
remember more or less meaningless things,
such as grammatical rules, it is possible to
learn them by making them into a kind of
doggerel verse, like that by which school-
boys learn Latin syntax. Provided that
somebody else has taken the trouble to
make the verse, it is easy to learn in this
way a large number of things that other-
wise would have to be learned mechanically
and so would be retained very uncertainly.

The most important factor of all in remembering is, however, the organisation of
our minds by previously acquired knowledge.
All that one has learned before on any
subject forms a kind of system of pigeon-
holing in the mind, by means of which new
knowledge can be fitted in. This has been
called the mind's " apperceptive system."

The mind is often spoken of as if it were
a bag or a room which can only contain a
certain number of things. It is suggested
that we should not try to learn too many
things lest the mind should become over-
crowded. This is an example of the misleading use of an analogy. The relationship

of the mind to its memories is something like that of a bag to its contents. It differs from it, however, in just this respect, that the more you put into a bag, the less room is there for other things, while the opposite is true of the mind. The greater the store of memories in the mind, the greater is its power of acquiring new ones. The man who has learnt one science finds it easier to learn another, for there is more knowledge in his mind with which his new knowledge can be related. In the same way the man who knows two languages finds it easier to learn a third, while the man who knows three languages finds it easier to learn a fourth, and so on.

This fact, that the more knowledge the mind has the more it can acquire, is one that cannot satisfactorily be expressed by any analogy. It is altogether obscured by comparing the mind with a bag. I tried a little earlier to express something of the truth by comparing the mind with a system of pigeon-holes. Even that, however, does not express the whole truth, for the papers you put on your shelves do not form themselves into pigeon-holes for the reception of yet more papers. Something like this is, however, true of the mind. It is the memories stored in the mind which make the system of filing and pigeon-holing for new memories; and, as these new memories are added, they too increase the capacity of the pigeon-holing system for yet more knowledge.

It is for this reason that those who have acquired, let us say, a large amount of knowledge about human anatomy or about the religion of Early Greece or about the history of the Pharaohs, will find themselves ready to retain with ease new bits of information about these same subjects. A great part of education is directed towards giving children usefully organised apperceptive systems in a wide variety of subjects about which they will have to learn more later. A boy who has learned electricity and magnetism at school may have learned very little of the actual instruments he will have to use if later he becomes an electrical engineer. He will, however, be able to learn these things, while the boy who knows no electricity will not. The first boy has an electrical apperceptive system while the second has not.

Suppose that anyone wants to learn a new subject, let us say psychology or economics.

155

He will soon be discouraged by finding that a great part of all the books he reads will be difficult to understand, and those which are so simply written that he cannot fail to understand them, he will find himself unable to remember. The extraordinary rapidity with which we find ourselves forgetting it, is one of the most disconcerting parts of trying to learn a new subject. Yet we should not allow ourselves to be discouraged at this stage. This forgetting does not mean that our brains are not adequate to cope with this subject, but simply that we have not yet formed an apperceptive system in which to receive it. We are putting papers on shelves which are not yet pigeon-holed to receive them.

Moreover, what you are reading is not lost although you cannot recall it. It is itself forming the apperceptive system for new knowledge (here, as we have seen, our analogy with the papers on the shelves breaks down).

It has been said that what is of value to you in learning a subject is not the small amount of it you remember, but the large amount of it you have forgotten. There is a great deal of truth in this, although perhaps " forgotten " is not quite the right word. The fact that we cannot recall something at will, does not mean necessarily that it is forgotten in the sense of being really lost to the mind. It may have become part of the permanent structure of the mind which makes new acquisitions of knowledge possible.

A last point about remembering which may be noticed is that the importance of precise remembering has been altered very much by the discovery a few thousand years ago of the art of writing. Some people who make a fetish of accurate and detailed remembering seem to have overlooked the practical usefulness of this discovery. In the days before the art of writing was discovered, knowledge was handed down from one generation to another by learning by heart what was told by the elders, and if a fact was not remembered in any mind the knowledge of it was gone for ever. Then accurate mechanical remembering was of great importance. Now, however, a fact you have written down and carefully filed, is as much your permanent possession as one that can be recalled out of your head, and it is better for most purposes to use writing than to rely on mental remembering for retaining a fact. There are few scientists who do not use filing systems to retain with precision the facts that they want to use in their writings.

WHEN we are lying asleep at night, our muscles are relaxed and we no longer respond by action to any call which may come to us from the outside world through our sense organs. Nor do we respond by action to the stimulations of the sense organs inside our own bodies. Lack of moisture inside the mouth may give rise to thirst. Instead, however, of going to the tap to get some water as we should if we were awake, our muscles remain relaxed.

Instead of external activity, there is a peculiar activity of our minds we call dreaming. We may dream simply that we have got up and gone to the tap to satisfy our thirst, or we may produce a more elaborate and picturesque dream of plunging into cool mountain streams or drinking deep flagons of foaming beer. Our minds have created a vivid drama of satisfying our thirst which seems to us sufficiently real to relieve us of the necessity for that external action which is actually required but which would cut short our sleep.

Like all purely mental activity, however, dreaming has the disadvantage of producing no real external results. The physical dryness causing the thirst continues in spite of the dream of quenching it. The dryness may, in the end, grow so strong that its demands can no longer be put off by mere dreaming about drinking. It will then stir us to actual action, which means that it will wake us up.

In the same way, when our landlady knocks on the bedroom door in the morning, we may dream that we are sitting in a park listening to a band in which the drummer is sounding a long tattoo, or, perhaps, that we hear a knocking on our bedroom door and that we are getting up and dressing. In either case, the dream is a fairly transparent attempt of our sleeping minds to evade real activity. In the first example, this is done by representing the noise as something which calls for no action on our part; in the second the mind recognises the knocking as a demand for activity but substitutes a dream activity for a real one. In both cases the dream is an attempted evasion of real action; it is trying to preserve sleep.

There are, of course, much more complicated disturbers of sleep than the simple ones which have just been described. The driving forces behind our waking activity are such things as our desire to win money, or fame, or somebody's love, or to provide security for our families. The incomplete satisfaction of such desires in our waking life may produce anxieties which will be serious sleep disturbers if our minds cannot lay them to rest during sleep by efficient dream formation. The restlessness of unsatisfied desire which makes it a serviceable spur to action in waking life, makes it also an enemy of sound sleep. If the acquisitiveness of the business man or the sense of frustration of the lover persist in their own forms during the night, their result will be light sleep, bad dreams, and insufficient rest.

If the mind does its dream-work effectively, however, sleep is undisturbed by unsatisfied desires. The business man achieves success in his dreams, the ambitious man is surrounded by the marks of other people's esteem, and the lover sleeps in the arms of his beloved. Then sleep is deep, and efficient rest repairs the fatigue of the day. It is not until morning that the restlessness and emptiness of unfulfilled desire return again to act as spurs to effective action.

The dream way of responding to demands for action is not, however, confined to sleep. Even during our waking hours, the formation of day-dreams or phantasies is part of our mental life. While these are not identical with the dreams of sleep, they are produced in the same general way. They are dramas of fulfilled desire. In our day-dreams, our ambitions are fulfilled, we win the esteem of other people and the affections of those we love, we carry out actions in which our physical or mental limitations are overcome, and we transport ourselves from the depressing industrial towns in which we are forced to earn our living and recreate ourselves on the mountains or sunlit sea-shore which our hearts desire. This is all, however, without immediate real effects on the outside world.

We may say, in fact, that there are two ways in which we can respond to any situation or feeling which impels us towards action. We may really act or we may dream. The clerk who realises that his salary is too small to enable him to marry may study a foreign language in order to

164

fit himself for a better-paid post, or he may be content just to picture himself in a position of responsibility. The student who realises that he does not know enough of his subject to pass his examinations may study his subject more diligently, or he may construct a phantasy of himself passing with first-class honours and receiving his degree before an admiring audience. On the side of actual activity, there is the advantage that it alone can produce real results; on the side of dreaming, there is that aversion to the hardships of real activity which is to be found in even the most energetic characters.

Nothing can be more fatal to the achievement of any ambition than this substitution of dreaming for real activity. It is a constant danger of all systems of mental culture that they are liable to encourage the dreaming rather than the acting habit of mind. There is a system which asks its students how long in each day they spend in thinking of their ambition, and implies that they ought to spend at least an hour a day in such thought. I think this is a dangerous question. A better question would be " How long in each day do you spend in actual activity towards realising your ambition? "

The clerk whose thoughts were occupied with his dream of becoming a managing director while he was engaged in adding up figures might easily find that his dismissal for incompetence took him further from the fulfilment of his ambition than he was before.

Such systems remind us that no change in the condition of a single individual or of society as a whole has ever been brought about unless it has first been imagined by somebody. That is true, and it alone would be sufficient reason for refusing to regard dreams as unimportant. There is, however, another truth which is liable to be overlooked. So long as a change remains merely imagined by someone and is not translated into action it is without real effects. It remains a mere dream.

You will do very little for the mitigation of poverty by giving a shilling to a man in distress, but even that little will be far more than will result from your merely dreaming that you have reorganised society from top to bottom. Such dreams are valuable and necessary, but only if they are translated into some effective action, however little it may accomplish.

In the early days of the great war some

people met together to " will " peace. They proposed to take no action, but were supported by a vague belief that mental conditions translated themselves into physical realities without any efforts being made to that end. It was a mere dream and not a " will " that they were producing, and any action, however trivial, would have had more real outside effects.

Just as dreaming of action is not acting, so dreaming of knowledge is not knowing. Since study is a hard kind of action many people are willing to substitute dreaming of knowledge for real learning. Hence the attraction of a certain kind of popular manual on scientific subjects in which difficulties are evaded, uncertainties and exceptions to accepted rules are forgotten, and the reader is led to believe that no more arduous discipline of thought is necessary to fit us to make an intelligent judgment on a scientific theory than that needed for solving magazine puzzles. The reading of such manuals bears to real learning about the same relationship as being pulled along a valley by a train bears to the arduously won joy of adventure on the mountain tops. The heights of science are open to some extent to everyone who has time to devote to study and who is not feeble-minded, but they are open to no one (not even to the most gifted) without mental discipline and hard work.

The science of psychology suffers in particular from such substitutes for real learning. So we find many people who feel able to give a just and final judgment on such questions as psycho-analysis, the existence and nature of human instincts, and modern theories of education with no more knowledge of these questions than they have acquired from their daily papers.

Simple manuals serving as introductions to difficult branches of knowledge are not, of course, in themselves harmful. These are often written by men eminent in research in their own subjects. Sir William Bragg's lectures on electrons and atoms can interest the person entirely ignorant of physics, but they would never lead him to suppose that a full understanding of this subject could be attained by such an easy path. They would be more likely to supply him with the interest which would stimulate him to the effort necessary for more advanced study of the subject. A person possessing the true spirit of the mountaineer but ignorant of the ways of mountains might begin by being led by a guide up easy slopes. He would never, however, make his acquaintance with the mountains by being drawn in a donkey cart through the valleys.

The temptation to substitute dreaming of knowledge for the real activity necessary to gain it is one that remains at all stages of learning. It is always easier to spin ingenious theories out of one's own mind than to win them by the impartial study of hard facts. Many men who have started as earnest students of reality have lost their way in the dreamland of fanciful theorising. Perhaps all do to some extent, and those who have made the great contributions to human knowledge have simply been those who resisted this temptation most successfully.

Whole nations have forgotten to study reality and have developed an intellectual culture which has had for its science mere speculations unchecked by fact—dream knowledge instead of real science. The seven million tiny vessels traversing the body called *nadis*, the latent and sacred energy of *Kundalini*, and the *Astral body* are some of the " discoveries " of this dream science.

169

Probably the chief reason for the survival amongst ourselves of fragments of such fanciful learning is that belief in them serves both mental idleness and the desire to feel that we know more than other people. It is easier to acquire the jargon of the astral body than it is to learn the names and functions of the spinal nerves from an anatomical textbook. Also this jargon can be made to sound very impressive to ignorant people. The textbook will give us real knowledge, however—knowledge which can be checked by observation and experiment —while the other is nothing but dream knowledge.

It is not, however, only from the pre-scientific systems of the East that we can draw this shadowy imitation of real knowledge. Whenever in our search for knowledge we lean back in our arm-chairs and spin fancies from our minds instead of applying ourselves to the study of reality, we are weaving a similar dream of our own. Many books are published every year which are produced by no more arduous mental effort than this. They are very vague and very general and very dull, and because most of their readers cannot understand

170

what they mean, their authors think that they are "philosophical." There could be no more cruel abuse of a noble word than to call such mystification "philosophy." A true philosophy is one that is in close touch with reality.

The danger of dreaming, then, is that it produces no real results. This is not to say, however, that dreaming serves no good end. So long as dreams are kept in their right place and are not allowed to interfere with action, the ability to dream is of no less value than the ability to act.

It is true in a sense of every aim that we accomplish that it was a dream before it was an accomplished reality. Our ability to plan far into the future, and to carry out an arduous course of training in order to fit ourselves in the end for a desired position, depends on our ability first to dream and then to use our own efforts to convert those dreams into a reality. Slavery could not have been abolished in America if Lincoln and others had not first dreamed of a condition of society in which all men had legal freedom. Nor would it have been abolished if these men had not had the energy to make this dream into a reality.

So dreams are not always idle substitutes for action. They may be spurs to action. It is usual to give a special name to those dreams which lead to action and to call them *ideals*. A medical student who dreams of himself as a famous and successful surgeon may find that this dream provides the necessary incentive to make him apply himself hard to his work, which is often laborious and dull. This is an ideal, for it obviously serves a useful purpose in his life. If, however, his dream took the form of picturing himself as an operatic singer applauded for his wonderful tenor voice, this would clearly be a useless dream, however pleasant it might be to the student himself.

But even an ideal may degenerate into an idle dream if it is indulged in for its own sake. If the medical student sits in his arm-chair picturing himself as a successful surgeon when he ought to be studying a textbook on anatomy, he is indulging in an amusement as useless to action as if he were engaged in the operatic tenor dream.

Whenever we are engaged in a task which we are not compelled to do by somebody else, we shall find that we can help ourselves to do it by encouraging ourselves with the picture of what we hope to have accomplished at the end of it. Writing a book is, for example, such a task. But, since work is irksome while dreaming is easy and pleasant, we shall find it necessary many times a day to kick ourselves into actual activity instead of merely dreaming about the finished result.

Dreams, of course, may sometimes be worth while in themselves apart from any value as stimulants to action. A work of art is just a dream which has been given an external form so that its beauty can be communicated to other persons. Its value may simply lie in its beauty. All dreaming, even when it remains in the mind of the dreamer and is incommunicable to other people, has the same kind of value. Nothing that makes men happier can be without value. The mental pictures of green hills and sunshine which may lighten the drab day of the worker in a smoky industrial city have something of the same kind of value as Keats's *Ode to the Nightingale*. Even if our dreams served no useful purpose in action, we should be very much poorer without them.

Perhaps it is hardly necessary to say this,

173

for few of us are inclined to undervalue
dreams. Most of us are more inclined to
forget how little dreams can do unless they
are translated into actions. We like to
judge ourselves favourably because of our
fine intentions, when it is really our active
efforts to accomplish those intentions that
matter. To lose touch with reality and live
entirely in a world of our own beautiful
dreams is a form of insanity which ends in
a mental decay in which probably even those
dreams are lost. Effort on the plane of
reality is a price we must pay for the privilege
of sane and healthy dreaming. If our dreams
even begin to take the place which should
be occupied by reality we begin to become
ineffective. We are mentally only half alive.

ANYONE who reads the advertisements of systems of mental culture will notice what a very large number of them promise to cure their students of shyness, to give them self-confidence and a " magnetic " personality which will make it possible for them to dominate other persons. These advertisements may be illustrated with some such picture as that of a previously diffident clerk demanding, with his chin thrust out and his chest inflated, a rise in salary from his employer.

There is no doubt that the sense of inferiority is a very great evil for those who suffer from it. The shyness which results from it and the loss of self-confidence or even of self-respect destroy both efficiency and happiness. To be able to give some help to people who suffer in this way should be one of the aims of applied psychology.

We must feel much less sympathetic with the ambition merely to dominate other people. If psychology could turn us all into chin-thrusting, chest-thumping personalities, we should not be any better off, for there would be no one left to be dominated. The human race as a whole would certainly suffer, for such mental monstrosities could not be expected to get on with one another and would most likely exterminate each other in a few years.

Although excessive timidity and lack of self-confidence are obvious sources of inefficiency in all that part of the business of life which is concerned with our relations to other people, efficiency is not to be gained merely by learning to dominate others. We do not best move through a crowd of people by going forward in a straight line and pushing everyone else by brute force out of our way. A better method is one which combines pushing forward and giving way. We walk round some of the people who are in our way, and occasionally step back for someone moving in the opposite direction; we try to take advantage wherever we can of currents of people moving in the same direction as ourselves, adjusting our movements all the time both to the requirements of other people and to our own aim of getting to the other side. In this way, we get to our destination not only without causing annoyance to anyone else, but also more quickly and with much less trouble to ourselves than if we had taken no notice of other people but had just pushed them out of the way.

This is equally true of all that part of our life in which we are concerned with other people. However definitely we may have decided on our aims, the best way to attain them is not just by pushing straight forward and ignoring the requirements of other people. We have instincts both of *submission* and of *assertion*, and it is only by a balanced exercise of both that we can keep a harmonious and efficient relationship with the people with whom we have to deal. If we are the victims of a sense of inferiority which makes us too submissive, we shall never attain our goals, because we shall be pushed on one side by the more forceful personalities of those with whom we are competing. If, however, we are too assertive, we are likely also to miss our aim, for we shall arouse the active antagonism of other people, and cut ourselves off from the advantages of co-operation. There are not many things worth gaining which we can gain alone, without the active co-operation of our fellow men.

If we went to consult a doctor about a serious illness, it would be of no help to us that we had taken a correspondence course in the development of a dominating personality which enabled us to impose our will and our opinion on him. This would merely put us into a position in which we could not profit from the knowledge and experience of the doctor. If we died as a result, our survivors could more justly write on our tombstone *Here lies a pig-headed individual* than *Here lies a magnetic personality.*

It is equally true, of course, that the doctor would fall short of full usefulness to his patients if he lacked that element of character which enabled him to impose his opinion and his will on them. We all require a certain ability to dominate in some situations and a certain ability to submit in others.

Even when we admit this, however, it remains true that lack of self-confidence and excessive shyness are always unpleasant and may be a serious disability. No one who suffers from them can be satisfied with the efficiency of his mind. They are common (and perhaps unavoidable) in the period between childhood and adult life, but the normal person outgrows them as he leaves adolescence behind him. If he is so unfortunate as to find that he does not, what can he do about it?

First of all, we must notice that there is one kind of shyness which stands in a class by itself because it is found in nearly everybody to begin with. This is the lack of self-confidence which assails us when we first try to speak in front of an audience. This is probably a real instinct and is the timidity which prevents the ordinary member of a herd of wild animals from assuming the position of leader. In the wild condition it was a useful reaction because the most efficient hunting or fighting organisation is that herd in which the dominance of the herd leader is most unquestioned.

However useful this peculiarity of character may have been to our remote ancestors, it is a great nuisance to the man or woman who must begin to speak in public either for the advancement of some cause or in order to earn a living. If you are in this position, you can comfort yourself with the reflection that you are facing a difficulty which practically every public speaker has faced and overcome. It is a disability which mere habit will get rid of. There are examples of people who find that after years of public speaking, they are as nervous before an audience as they were when they began, but these are rare. Most people find that the habit of speaking before an audience makes it as easy to speak in that way as to carry on a conversation with their own friends.

This fact should prevent the nervous beginner in public speaking from being too much depressed by his nervousness, but it does not solve his immediate problem of how to get on until his nervousness disappears. The principles to be applied are the same as those described in an earlier chapter on the control of other emotions.

There is first the principle of the control of emotional expression. Even though you cannot by willed effort stop yourself from feeling timid in front of an audience, you can stop yourself from showing the outward signs of timidity. You can stop your knees from knocking together and your voice from quavering. If you can succeed in showing no outward sign of your feeling of nervousness at the beginning, half the battle is won, for your nervousness will rapidly grow less as you go on speaking.

If willed effort is not sufficient to keep down the outward signs of nervousness, auto-suggestion should be used. A short formula should be repeated saying that you will speak confidently and well, and (since too much anxiety about your speech is a great cause of your nervousness) that the whole business does not matter much. This last part of your formula can be quite properly used if (and only if) you have previously done every-thing you can by strenuous preparation to make your speech as good as it can be. Much of your nervousness would disappear if you could fully realise that the great course of the universe would be unaltered by the good or bad impression your speech made on the persons who heard it.

It will be found a good plan to repeat this formula several times during the few days just before the dreaded event, particularly when the thought of the intended speech is already making you feel nervous. It will be found helpful to form a mental picture of the audience as they will appear from the plat-form and to look them straight in the face while repeating the formula. It should also be repeated (silently, of course) immediately before speaking. You should look boldly round the audience before speaking, and at them while speaking. By the use of these methods it should be found that the fear of an audience can be effectively controlled.

A more difficult problem, however, faces the man who finds himself timid and lacking in self-confidence in all his contacts with other persons, and who finds that mere habit does nothing to remove his misfortune. He it is who is attracted by the advertisements which promise him a " magnetic personality " and the power of dominating other people. He suffers from what the psycho-analysts call an " inferiority complex."

The methods which have just been mentioned for the normal person overcoming his fear of speaking in public apply, of course, also to the man suffering from a real inferiority complex. He too must remember that he has a certain amount of control over the expression of his emotion of fear even though he has none over the emotion itself. A confident bearing with head held up and voice firm will both help to remove the inner lack of self-confidence and also hide it from other persons. The shy person will find help too in formulæ of auto-suggestion suggesting self-confidence, clear and unhesitating speech, and freedom from the inner doubts which assail him when he tries to influence other persons.

His danger here is what is technically known as *over-compensation*. If the practice of a self-confident voice and manner and the use of auto-suggestion merely change him from a shy and diffident man into an arrogant and self-assertive one, not much will have been gained. Arrogance does not help us in our relationships with other men any better than does timidity, and it is a much more unpleasant quality of character. This replacement of timidity by arrogance is just what is likely to happen as a result of the methods just described if no attempt is made to attack the deeper roots of the trouble.

Lack of self-confidence and timidity are merely surface results of a deep underlying doubt and under-valuation of ourselves. Auto-suggestion and the practice of a self-confident manner leave this doubt untouched, so instead of expressing our doubt of ourselves in timidity we try to hide it by an outward show of arrogance. The arrogance, however, is very unlike the calm self-reliance

185

of the man who has no doubts of himself. The voice tends to be too loud, and we are self-assertive when self-assertion is not necessary.

We do not need a training in psychology to recognise the difference between the man who is really self-confident and the man who puts on the manner of self-confidence in order to hide his deep-seated sense of inferiority. In just the same way, no sensible person supposes that the man who shows habitual foolhardiness in exposing himself to unnecessary danger is really (as he would like us to believe) a man in whom the sense of danger is absent. It is more likely that he indulges in these freaks as an over-compensation for a deep-seated fearfulness. We are not surprised if the same man shows utter cowardice in the presence of an unexpected and unavoidable danger.

It is for this reason that we have spoken of an *inferiority complex* and not merely of the feeling of inferiority. It is something more complicated than a mere feeling that the uncontrollably shy man is suffering from. Whether its outward expression is a timid manner, or a boastful manner, or a pompous manner, or an affected and " cultured " manner, the root trouble is the same. It is an inferiority complex expressing itself in various objectionable ways. The aim of the man suffering from the sense of inferiority should be to cure the disease which lies at the root of his trouble and not merely to change its symptom into one which may be even more objectionable than mere shyness.

Before we discuss how this can be done, we must notice the dangers and disadvantages of one of the specifics recommended for the domination of other persons. This is the copying of the methods used in hypnotism.

It is found that many people can be put into the hypnotic state and in that state can be made to do or believe whatever the hypnotiser wishes, by the use of methods which can obviously be imitated in everyday life. The hypnotiser looks straight into his patient's eyes and repeats his requirements over and over again in a calm, commanding, and monotonous voice. He does not argue or reason with his patient but simply commands. It was supposed at one time that the hypnotiser had to make a great effort of will in order to dominate his patient, until Galton discovered that no special effort of will was required, but that all the hypnotiser need do was to adopt a manner of speaking and acting which would suggest to his patient that he was exerting the irresistible force of an inflexible will. So he was able to dominate his patient with a completeness which might rouse the envy of the most successful street-corner seller of a worthless drug for curing all diseases.

Similar methods are, in fact, used by the street-corner seller. They are often used also by orators and by the more bullying kind of reputable salesmen. These people try to influence other people's actions for their own ends by loud-voiced and confident repetition without reason or argument, and, if they are dealing with a single person, by looking him straight in the eyes. Is this the method which psychology recommends to us as the best for attaining efficiency in our relationships with other persons?

The most important part of the answer to this question is that even if these methods were as successful as their advocates say they are, they would be morally wrong. It is no more justifiable to use mental violence against other persons than to use physical violence. The injury to a man which may result from this sort of violence may be no less than if we

188

had persuaded him to buy our goods or to subscribe to our creed by bashing him in the face until he did. The injury will show less because it is in his mind and not in his body.

I suggest that the circumstances in which these hypnotic tricks are justifiable are very rare indeed. Perhaps they are entirely confined to the doctor's consulting-room. There are very rare circumstances in which we are justified in using physical violence against another person. If we are rescuing a man from drowning and he clutches us in such a way that he is endangering the lives both of himself and his rescuer, we are justified in rendering him unconscious by a blow on the jaw. Circumstances of a similar kind are necessary to justify the use of hypnotic tricks for forcing your will on another person. The individual who uses them for selling a patent medicine or a metal polish should be locked up.

A further point to notice is that such methods are not always as successful as their advocates would have us believe. When dealing with a crowd, one can certainly produce greater immediate effects by confident repetition than by argument, but there is good reason for believing that effects produced in this way are not very lasting. Every member of a crowd is also an individual who will think over in solitude what he has heard. If it has been nothing but windy and empty repetition, it is not likely to appear very convincing to him as he reflects over it by his fireside, even if he was carried away at the time of hearing it.

The effects of using hypnotic tricks on an individual may be even less what the person using them expected. The subordinate who uses the hypnotic gaze and manner when asking his employer for a rise in salary may find that his employer has been studying the same book on applied psychology as himself. In that case, the applicant is likely to find himself kicked through the door instead of being promoted.

Even those people who know no psychology are generally provided by nature with a fairly efficient mechanism for protecting them against too unscrupulous attempts to overthrow the independence of their wills. Such attempts are likely to arouse the attitude of " contra-suggestion " or refusal to act in the way expected. A judge who is too positive in his directions to the jury may find that they bring in a verdict against his directions and against the evidence, simply because they were moved to an attitude of antagonism by his too obvious attempt to dictate to them. Similarly, a man may refuse to buy an article for no better reason than that, without knowing the technical name for the process, he has recognised that the seller is trying to influence his judgment by the kind of psychological trickery we have been describing.

I am frequently visited by people who want to sell me apparatus for the laboratory. Some of these have learnt their salesmanship in the hypnotic school, and they stare me down and talk in loud confident voices. They are at a loss, however, when I ask them about some technical detail of the apparatus. They believe that self-assertion is more important for a salesman than accurate knowledge. These are not the ones to whom I am most inclined to give orders, and I do not think that I am very different in this way from other people. If, in the business world, you can best sell things by loud-voiced self-assertion, then business men must be bigger fools than they are generally supposed to be.

Chapter XI   The Destruction of the Inferiority Complex

N

WE must return, however, to the problem of the methods of dealing with the root causes of the sense of inferiority. The person who suffers acutely from this may take some comfort from the fact that it is an affliction which to some extent nearly everyone has suffered from. The man who has always been naturally and completely without doubts of himself must be very rare. A haunting sense of inferiority is common at adolescence and immediately afterwards, but most people manage to deal with it satisfactorily at this time, while a few others carry the same affliction through the rest of their lives.

The beginning of it may lie in childhood. The foolish mother who says in her daughter's hearing " I wish Amelia had been a boy," or the foolish visitor who says " Now that your little baby brother is born, Mother won't love you any more," may sow in the child's mind a seed which will ripen into an inferiority complex from which he or she will never in later life be free. There are many crimes which are not punishable by law, but few more cruel than this one.

There may, on the other hand, be a more real cause for the development of a sense of inferiority in childhood. The child, for example, may be less beautiful or less intelligent than his brothers and sisters. The evil will, of course, be greater if the parents show preference for the others, but it may be there in any case. Or, there may be an actual bodily inferiority, a deformity or serious bodily weakness. Hunchbacks are proverbially liable to display the unpleasant traits of character which develop from an inferiority complex. Or the child may find himself looked down upon because he is of a race regarded as inferior by the majority of people amongst whom he lives, or because he is of mixed blood and is despised by the men and women of both races from which he has sprung.

There is no biological reason for the moral degeneracy often found amongst half-caste people. A man half Chinese and half English is not physically or mentally worse off than if he were of pure race. He may,

196

however, be mean and degraded simply because from childhood he has found himself despised alike by the Chinese and the English. In places where the half-caste is not despised he is not found to be mentally or morally inferior. There are, no doubt, real differences between people of different races, but we may well ask how much of the supposed inferiority of the races we believe to be inferior to ourselves may be due to a racial inferiority complex, produced by our triumphant attitude of superiority.

An inferiority complex may, then, have started in a humiliation of childhood the reality of which has long since passed away, or it may have its roots in a lifelong humiliation through bodily defect or membership of a despised race or caste. In either case we must deal with it as it exists at present. It is not wise to try by ourselves to dig out its roots in the distant past. This is what is done in the method of treatment known as psycho-analysis. This treatment under the direction of an expert analyst may sometimes be the right one for severe cases. It is, however, a long process and it is not one we can undertake by ourselves.

For those who are trying without outside

help to cure themselves, the advice undoubtedly is to leave the past alone and to fight the evil as it exists at present. It is the present under-valuation of yourself that is at fault, and the only method is to drag this under-valuation into the clear limelight of consciousness and to destroy it by understanding it, by laughing at it, and by refusing to accept it any more.

It is not being a hunchback or having a coloured skin that makes you feel inferior. It is not even the fact that other people think less of you for these things. It is your accepting the valuation of other people and despising yourself that is the real trouble. This is what you must not allow.

Those who have any tendency to undervalue themselves but who have no ground for it in a supposed bodily or racial inferiority find rich material for the creation of an inferiority complex in customary social valuations. The desire to associate with the rich and idle; embarrassment in their presence because our manner of dressing, eating, and speaking are not the same as theirs; or even loud assertion of our equality with them, are all marks of the acceptance of a superstition which must be cast out if we wish to be free from the sense of inferiority.

In their hearts, most people must recognise that the fictions of social position are superstitions more worthy of savages than of thinking people. Yet the whole system is often so worked into the stuff of their minds that many persons prefer any folly, unhappiness or embarrassment to a courageous repudiation of it.

Why, for example, should a man be tortured with embarrassment because he is conscious of being dressed differently and of handling his knife and fork differently from the prosperous-looking man at the next table? He does not reflect that the prosperous-looking man might as sensibly be embarrassed because his own dress and manners are not the same as his neighbour's. These conventions differ in different places and there is no absolute standard of right and wrong. The prosperous man maintains (very sensibly) the fiction that his conventions are absolutely right, while his shy neighbour has foolishly accepted the same fiction.

The remedy for an inferiority complex must often be to remove from the mind the fictitious valuations of caste. The shop-assistant who looks down on the general servant is accepting a system of judgments by which she is logically led to accept the typist's similar under-valuation of herself. We cannot accept a system which leads us to despise others without being in danger of being led by it to despise ourselves, and it is this despising of ourselves (unrecognised by consciousness) which is an inferiority complex. If we are to keep our respect for ourselves, we cannot afford to allow ourselves the luxury of thinking ourselves superior to others who follow different occupations, who have differently coloured skins, or even who have less intelligence.

If we realise that this deep-rooted under-valuation of ourselves is at the root of our inferiority complexes, the general rules for dealing with these will be clear. We must undertake a thorough revision of our attitude towards ourselves and towards other people. Controlled thinking will help us to this end. Science, religion and common-sense will all provide reflections which will help us to win a sane outlook on ourselves and on other people.

No one who has fully realised the position

of the human race clinging precariously for a little time to a globe hurtling through space, with no protection against collision with one of the multitude of other globes, will feel unduly lifted up by the fact that he has a superior social position or depressed because he hasn't. The varying gifts which separate individuals will seem small too to one who fully realises the long process of evolution which has gone to the making of man. What a long and laborious process was the making of the backbone in the vertebrate animals. The hunchback may reflect that to have a backbone at all is a finer thing than merely to have one that is straight, and a man may certainly be prouder of having a skin than merely of having one without colouring matter in it.

So we can all cultivate a pride in the things we have in common with all men, and only allow ourselves a very small allowance of satisfaction in the gifts which are peculiar to ourselves. We cannot hope to get rid of this satisfaction altogether and, in any case, it is of use to temper the inferiority we may be led to feel in the superior gifts of others. All of us are peculiarly gifted in some respects, and it is foolish always to put ourselves into positions in which our inferiorities are too obvious to ourselves. If we are not good-looking, we may be good speakers, and if we are not good speakers we may have a fine sense of humour. If we are no good at football, we may have a rare gift for tiddly-winks; so we shall be wise not always to be trying to play football but sometimes to allow ourselves to display our gifts at tiddly-winks. We ought to play football as well for the sake of our humility. It is neither pride nor humility that we are aiming at, but at a serviceable balance between the two.

While practising such a discipline of thought and behaviour in order to get rid of the inferiority complex in all of its forms and to attain real freedom in our relation-ships with other men, we can, of course, use auto-suggestion in order to relieve the dis-tressing symptoms of shyness, etc., when they occur. The student who is suffering from stage fright at the prospect of a viva-voce examination to-morrow cannot wait until his views of his relation to his fellow men have improved before he escapes from his paraly-sing shyness. He must have relief now, and his method will be to use auto-suggestion as described in the last chapter. Only he should remember that he is merely giving relief to a symptom and not curing the disease.

Another thing that may be wrong with a person suffering from an inferiority complex is that he is unnaturally engrossed in what other people are thinking about him. We are all sensitive to other people's opinion to some extent, and it is right that we should be. But if we are always suffering at the thought of their real or imaginary disapproval of our behaviour or of our dress, then we must recognise this habit and destroy it as we destroy other bad habits.

When we have properly subdued our inferiority complexes, we shall not, of course, show our independence of other people's opinions by discarding our collars and spitting on the pavements. Such a vigorous rebellion against harmless conventions does not show that one is really free from them, but suggests that one has an inner slavery to them against which one is kicking. The man really free from slavery to the opinions of others will conform to conventions which do no harm and reserve his opposition for the many customary ways of behaving and feeling which are cruel, inefficient and harmful.

MOST of the systems of mental self-development which we have been discussing have been parts of the practice of religious systems. That is clearly not just an accident. Part of the driving force behind man's ceaseless quest for religion has been his need for the development of an attitude and a system of beliefs in which his restlessness and his fears, his worries and his inefficiencies may disappear.

The deepest and most essential part of the faith of all religions is the conviction that our business is to identify ourselves with a purpose infinitely more important than any of our private ends. This purpose is what the religious man calls " the Will of God." In this phrase, the word God has been used in the most widely different senses. By most religious men God has been believed in as a personal Being; others, however, have thought of Him only as an impersonal force. His Will also has been differently understood,

207

and the conception of it has varied from the ruthless massacre of unbelievers to the establishment of justice, kindness, and equality of opportunity for all men.

However it may be believed in, it is evident that a real acceptance of the Will of God lifts the religious man from the region of worries and fears. One who truly feels himself as part of an infinite purpose cannot worry about his own failures, for he believes that his own efforts are only part of a process which can go on without them, and that although his efforts may be directed towards God's ends, God can work towards these ends by other means as well.

I have suggested in earlier chapters reflections which can be used to reduce the strength of particular emotions. The religious man will draw many others from his religious faith. The conception of all men as children of God should be enough to destroy unreasonable anger against other persons, or pride of race and all the other emotions connected with complexes of superiority and inferiority. In the same way, religious considerations should be found strong enough to remove all attitudes of worry and anxiety.

We must not, however, make the mistake

of supposing that the objects of the teachers of religion are the same as those of the mental culturist. In a sense they are opposites. The religious teacher tries to persuade men to believe in God and to take a religious attitude towards their conflicts and losses. He then shows that, having this faith, they must release themselves from the worries and fears which are inconsistent with it. He does not tell them to believe in God because they may so escape from their worries and fears, but that they must abandon their worries and fears because they believe in God.

Jesus taught his disciples not to worry because they saw how God took care even of the birds and the flowers. A mental culturist might invert this teaching and tell people to apply psychological methods to induce a belief that there was a God who took care of the birds and flowers, because in this way they could get rid of worry. This, however, would be to try to buy the consolations of religious faith at the price of mental dishonesty.

Whatever particular beliefs a religious man holds, it will be through these that he strives for mental efficiency. Also we may notice that if the religious attitude of mind is accepted, mental efficiency is no longer a low or utilitarian ideal. If we were only busy with our own ends it would matter to no one but ourselves whether we pursued them efficiently or not. But if there is an Eternal purpose which we can help or hinder by our actions, then it becomes of infinite importance how effective our action is. Mental efficiency becomes a religious duty.

It is a common error to associate especially with religion, those kinds of activity which are ineffective. The useless action of giving a penny to a beggar is supposed to be an act of religious charity, while religion is supposed to have nothing particular to do with an economic study of the causes of poverty and with political action to remove those causes. Yet these may be effective actions, while the first certainly is not.

In the same way, bathing the wounds of an injured person (which may be a dangerous operation for him if the water is not properly sterilised) is thought of as a religious act, while the scientific research and the medical organisation which make effective healing possible are not.

It is true that giving a penny to a beggar may be a religious act because it is done for the love of God. But there is something wrong with our religion if the love of God cannot also drive us to the effective action of economic research and political action.

So we ought not to regard as specially religious those types of mental activity and those organisations of mind which are inefficient. The religious man should not tolerate in himself the vague benevolence and general ineffectiveness which lead to no serviceable action. Mental inefficiency is an offence against the God whose instruments we are.

www.ingramcontent.com/pod-product-compliance
Lightning Source LLC
Chambersburg PA
CBHW031431270326
41930CB00007B/654